Home Long-Term Oxygen Treatment in Italy

The Additional Value of Telemedicine

R.W. Dal Negro • A.I. Goldberg (Eds)

Home Long-Term Oxygen Treatment in Italy

The Additional Value of Telemedicine

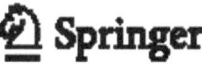 Springer

R.W. DAL NEGRO, MD, FCCP
Lung Department
Bussolengo General Hospital
Bussolengo (Verona), Italy
Vice-President
Italian Society of Respiratory Medicine (SIMeR)

A.I. GOLDBERG, MD, MBA, FAAP, FACPE, Master FCCP
Professor of Pediatrics
Loyola University Chicago, USA
Past-President, American College of Chest Physicians
Past-President, American Academy of Home Care Physicians

The Editors and Authors wish to thank VitalAire Italia Spa,
in particular Dr. Roberto Erba, for their contribution to this book

Library of Congress Control Number: 2005934784

ISBN 10   88-470-0388-1   Springer Milan Berlin Heidelberg New York
ISBN 13   978-88-470-0388-0

Springer is a part of Springer Science+Business Media
springeronline.com
© Springer-Verlag Italia 2005
Printed in Italy

The use of general descriptive names, registered names, trademarks,etc. in this publication does not imply, even in the absence of a specific statement, that such names are exempt from the relevant protective laws and regulations and therefore free for general use.
Product liability: The publishers cannot guarantee the accuracy of any information about dosage and application contained in this book. In every individual case the user must check such information by consulting the relevant literature.

Cover design: Massimiliano Caleffi
Typesetting: Marco Lorenti
Printing: Lineadue, Marnate (VA)

Preface

As an American, I recently began extending visits to friends in Italy by meeting families providing "agriturismo". My Italian speaking wife Evi (Eveline Faure, MD, FCCP, a graduate of the *Università Italiana per Stranieri*, Perugia) made this possible.

During one visit in 1994, we were sitting around the table in Pisa with friends who were fellow critical care physicians. They were remarking how specialists needed more patients. We told them that we were going south beyond Naples, a concept which they could not understand, considering the beauty of Tuscany. We had a marvelous time in southern Italy, meeting warm and welcoming people, surely one of the greatest resources of all Italy.

While in Calabria, I noted there were so many people on the streets joyfully communicating on their cell phones. (This was before cellular technology became so popular in the USA). Evi commented how tele-communication had advanced in Italy; she remembered how it took three hours to make a phone call with a jetton only a few years before. Later, in a small town (Revello, Basilicata), we met a wonderful young family who told us how difficult it was to get medical care. Yes, they had good general physicians, but it was hard to reach specialists many kilometers away. At the time, we were staying on a farm with an elderly couple, who invited us to join them to share meals. During conversation, I learned that the farmer had chronic lung disease and required long-term oxygen. He, too, found it difficult to get the care he needed in rural Italy.

I started to think... specialists up North, need in the South ... why not connect by tele-communication??

Many years later, I was introduced to telemedicine. As I traced its world-wide evolution, I was given a trade association report (un-authored) about a well-established program in Verona that used telemedicine for long-term oxygen management of chronic respiratory illness. I included this observation during a Memorial Lecture to honor the late Luciano Pesce, MD, FCCP, in Padua several years later. In the audience sat a gentleman who smiled as I did. Later, he introduced himself to me as Roberto Dal Negro, MD, FCCP. He humbly noted to me that he was grateful that I have acknowledged his team's work in Verona!

I have followed with admiration the work of Dott. Dal Negro and colleagues in

Veneto ever since. Their extensive experience with outcome analysis is an important demonstration of the value of telemedicine in home care. It would interest all those involved with long-term care for chronic illness (physicians, patients and families, health care organizations and funders, public policy leaders etc.) in Italy and elsewhere. This book is an effort to extend the awareness of their major accomplishment so all can understand the benefit to patients and families around the world.

Allen I. Goldberg
Professor of Pediatrics
Loyola University Chicago, USA
Past-President, American College of Chest Physicians
Past-President, American Academy of Home Care Physicians

Contents

Contributors

S. Amaducci
Department of Pneumology
San Carlo Borromeo Hospital
Milan, Italy

E. Battaglia
Department of Pneumology
San Carlo Borromeo Hospital
Milan, Italy

R. Bisato
Lung Department
Bussolengo General Hospital
Bussolengo (Verona), Italy

R. Cadinu
Lung Department
Bussolengo General Hospital
Bussolengo (Verona), Italy

D. Colombo
Respiratory Department
Pulmonary Rehabilitation Unit
INRCA - Scientific Institute
Casatenovo (Lecco), Italy

R.W. Dal Negro
Lung Department
Bussolengo General Hospital
Bussolengo (Verona), Italy

F. Facchini
Lung Department
Bussolengo General Hospital
Bussolengo (Verona), Italy

M. Farina
EmmeEffe, Management & Formazione
Milan, Italy

A. Fumagalli
Respiratory Department
Pulmonary Rehabilitation Unit
INRCA - Scientific Institute
Casatenovo (Lecco), Italy

M. Gaiani
IT Business Department, ALS
VitalAire Spa
Milan, Italy

A.I. Goldberg
Professor of Pediatrics
Loyola University
Chicago, USA

E.E. Guffanti
Respiratory Department
Pulmonary Rehabilitation Unit
INRCA - Scientific Institute,
Casatenovo (Lecco), Italy

C. Guglielmetti
IT Business Department, ALS
VitalAire Spa
Milan, Italy

C. Lucioni
Wolters Kluwer Health
Adis International ltd.
Milan, Italy

C. Micheletto
Lung Department
Bussolengo General Hospital
Bussolengo (Verona), Italy

C. MISURACA
Respiratory Department
Pulmonary Rehabilitation Unit
INRCA - Scientific Institute
Casatenovo (Lecco), Italy

P. PESCATORI
Lung Department
Bussolengo General Hospital
Bussolengo (Verona), Italy

S. TOGNELLA
Lung Department
Bussolengo General Hospital
Bussolengo (Verona), Italy

F. TREVISAN
Lung Department
Bussolengo General Hospital
Bussolengo (Verona), Italy

C. TURATI
Lung Department
Bussolengo General Hospital
Bussolengo (Verona), Italy

P. TURCO
PhD, University of Milan, Italy

R. RAVASIO
Wolters Kluwer Health
Adis International ltd.
Milan, Italy

A. VIGANÒ
Informatic Engineer
Cassano Magnano, Varese, Italy

Introduction

Home long-term oxygen treatment (H-LTOT) has evolved a great deal over the last years and represents an important advance in the treatment of diseases involving chronic respiratory insufficiency. However, little has been done in the past 20 years to refine or extend the results of early clinical trials, and there is remarkably little current research in this area.

The objective of administering LTOT is to cure hypoxemia and improve the patient's life expectancy and quality. Recommendations for using this technology are clearly specified in the scientific literature and there is a consensus of opinion among most of the professionals involved, although in many situations its clinical application does not follow the recommendations on its practice.

Moreover, we still do not know the efficacy of LTOT in patients with moderate resting hypoxemia, the efficacy of LTOT in patients who are normoxic when awake and at rest but who desaturate during physical activity or sleep, the optimal timing and dosage of oxygen supplementation, the mechanisms of action, the clinical and biochemical predictors of responsiveness to LTOT, or methods for enhancing adherence to LTOT. These questions need rapid responses, but it is really difficult to give the right answers if the patient must be treated at home for a very long period.

Telemedicine is a useful way to provide consultation-liaison services in the primary care setting. Telemedicine or better, telemonitoring, is defined as the use of information technology to monitor patients at a distance. The most promising applications for telemonitoring are to allow home monitoring of chronic illnesses such as cardiopulmonary disease, asthma, and heart failure. Telemonitoring allows reduction of chronic disease complications thanks to a better follow-up, provides health care services without using hospital beds, and reduces patient travel, time off from work, and overall costs. Several systems have proven to be cost effective. Telemonitoring is also a way of responding to the new needs of home care in an ageing population.

The possibility of also using telemonitoring in H-LTOT is extremely interesting. In fact, it could potentially offer several of the necessary solutions and surely limit the inconveniences. This book, edited by Roberto W. Dal Negro and Allen I. Goldberg, gives us a full account of the impact of the telemedicine system on H-LTOT. According to the information in this book, we have to begin to think about the possibility of using telemonitoring in H-LTOT in a really general manner. In fact, telemonitoring allows better control of the compliance of patients suffering from respiratory failure, and this means a better clinical condition and longer survival, both linked to the long-term administration of oxygen. Moreover, it also permits a reduction in expenditure for the management of patients under LTOT. Obviously, the general use of telemedicine in the evaluation of H-LTOT could meet with resistance from both physicians and patients, which could occur due to lack of correct information. However, I am sure that the in-depth reading of this book will reduce much of this resistance.

I am also sure that in the future, virtual reality, immersive environments, haptic feedback and nanotechnology will provide new ways to improve the capabilities of telemonitoring. However, acceptance in routine clinical practice could be hindered because of "human factors" or "man-machine interface" problems. Generally speaking, it seems that for the general population, Internet and mobile technology is viewed positively nowadays, and the benefits gained have already begun to be recognized by the doctors. Physicians represent one of the principal groups of telemedicine users and their acceptance of this technology constitutes one of the prerequisites to the emergence and sustainability of telemedicine networks. However, the decision of physicians to adopt a new technology such as telemedicine can be challenged by their relatively low computer literacy, the possible alteration of their traditional routines, and their high professional autonomy. It is clear that physicians must be given adequate information on the role of telemedicine systems in provision of health care, operational and support policies must be adequately developed and cost versus benefit of use must be clearly demonstrated.

It has been recently affirmed (Celli and colleagues) that technology will not replace patient care; it is merely a tool to make us more efficient. I completely agree with them. In any case, I also think that medical practice requirements should drive technology acquisition. Maximizing new technology to improve medical practices is certainly an objective of this plan, but functional medical needs must ultimately drive the acquisition of technology if the plan is to be successful. Considering this challenge, I am sure that telemedicine has a real additional value in H-LTOT.

Mario Cazzola
Unit of Pneumology and Allergology
Department of Respiratory Medicine
A. Cardarelli Hospital
Naples, Italy

Telemedicine in Respiratory Care

A.I. Goldberg

A Future Vision for the Use of Telemedicine in Respiratory Care

Telemedicine. What is it? Who uses it? When can it be useful? Where has it been used? Why is it important? How can it make a difference in delivering long-term care at home? Can it improve access to specialty care to improve health and overcome disparities? These and other questions may need answers in the mind of the reader.

This chapter will attempt to introduce "telemedicine" from multiple perspectives and for multiple purposes. It will briefly review some recent past uses in the home for respiratory care and then provide evidence from present experiences. To understand a future scenario from the present situation, current universal trends will be described from a global perspective. Then a preferred scenario (future vision) will be described to justify more universal acceptance and utilization of telemedicine in the care of patients, provision of services, and education of health care professionals and patients that will foster communication, collaboration, and a care partnership between patients and physicians.

What is "Telemedicine" (e-Health)?

The definition of telemedicine depends on the perspective of its users and its purposes.

A "technological" definition of telemedicine is the use of telecommunication technologies to exchange health information and provide health care services across geographic, temporal, social, and cultural barriers [1]. Technologies described range from plain telephone/fax communication through web-based computer applications that store/forward or provide real-time connectivity, to providing advanced virtual reality techniques. Such technologies facilitate interactive communication of data, text, audio, video and digital imaging. From a clinician's perspective, telemedicine is a mode of health care delivery that permits diagnosis, consultation, treatment, transfer of medical information and education, utilizing interactive video, visual, and data communication [2].

A public health view describes the functions of telemedicine as "removing distance and time barriers via technology in the provision of health services and health information" [3].

The Institute of Medicine of the National Academy of Sciences described telemedicine as "the use of electronic information and communication technology to provide and support health care when distances separate the participants" [4]. The IOM report described multiple clinical applications, including use for:

1. initial urgent evaluation: triage, stabilization, transfer, and disposition of patients requiring immediate acute attention
2. supervision of primary care by non-physicians or in the absence of a physician
3. one-time/continuing provision of specialty care when specialists are not available
4. consultation, including second-opinions
5. monitoring of patients as part of follow-up care in chronic disease management
6. remote information/decision analysis to support/guide care for specific patients.

Telemedicine has great potential to provide emergency, primary and specialty health care as well as education of health care professionals and patients/familes across time and space barriers. The integrated electronic transfer of information can have even greater impact since it can be collected, evaluated, and disseminated for clinical outcomes, evidence-based research, health services management (quality/cost management) and public policy formulation (health care finance). The value for patient and family health has been recognized especially with chronic disease management. The concepts of "telemedicine" have been broadened to "telehealth" and "e-health". This has been a response, in part, to patient/family demand for more access to reliable health information and promotion of telemedicine to improve health by patient education and self-management. In addition, electronic access to information has been used to improve patient-physician communication as a collaborative partnership. The notion that providing education and information to patients should be integral to promoting health has led to the concepts of "information therapy" and "information prescription" [5,6].

The Past: How has Telemedicine Been Used Recently to Provide Respiratory Care?

Telemedicine in general has been used to extend multiple specialty consultations and health services across geographic regions with limited access to health care. Thus, it has extended access to care in rural and remote areas by providing connectivity to major centres that can monitor and manage clinical needs for emergent, acute, and chronic health needs. Telemedicine has had strategic application in metropolitan areas, within and across broader geographic regions (states, provinces, countries) and internationally, to provide care, extend care to alternative settings (home and mobile care) and integrate health care system operations and management. Telemedicine has facilitated interactive information exchange for clinical and administrative purposes and permitted enhanced communication and education for health care professionals and patients/families.

The Italian experience for over a quarter of a century with long-term oxygen management in the home of chronic respiratory disease patients is of major significance. This is because, in contrast to applications in other medical/surgical specialties, telemedicine experience in respiratory care has been limited. However, there have been a few good examples of focused programs that have demonstrated value in respiratory/chronic care:

1. *Tele-education in asthma*: enhancing rural access/outreach and education to high-risk patients. Providing patient education in the proper use of medication and inhaler techniques resulting in improved patient knowledge and satisfaction for asthma self-management [7].

2. *Tele-monitoring/management of sleep disorders*: improved access to specialist care and reduced costs to patients with sleep disorders in remote areas. Featuring polysomnography and alternative diagnostic procedures (on-line transfer from remote rural sites) as well as remote monitoring data transfer to specialty centers for scoring and interpretation. Useful for diagnosis, determination of clinical severity, and management of treatment [8].

3. *Tele-interpretation of spirometry*: medical center specialty/technical support of remote site pulmonary function testing for earlier interventions and reduced misinterpretations [9].

4. *Care coordination for chronic health management*: case management by advanced practice nurses and social workers using tele-monitoring and in-home message devices, disease management tools, computers with chat rooms resulting in reduced hospitalizations and emergency room visits, improved clinical outcomes and patient satisfaction, improved access and reduced cost [10].

5. *Patient education for chronic health management*: providing health education and tele-communication with primary care providers for education and empowering patients to adopt preventative measures and healthy behaviors. Permitting patient self-management and maintaining more individuals with chronic disease in the community [11].

6. *Rural outpatient pulmonary care*: extending pulmonary specialty care from a major urban medical center 450 miles (700 km) from rural hospitals, providing pre- and post-procedural evaluations resulting in saving travel time and money and increasing access to pulmonary consultation [12].

7. *Specialty e-consultations*: access by remote physicians to medical center specialist with guaranteed e-mail response within 24 hours of request [13].

Telemedicine has proven value for long-term management of home respiratory care. Videophones for patients requiring mechanical ventilation in the home have permitted monitoring by the critical care specialists who discharged them from the ICU to home [14]. Respiratory care specialists support primary care physicians and families, reducing the number of house calls, unscheduled hospital visits and hospital admissions. This reduces the number of hours of unscheduled medical care and relieves family anxiety as specialist time is more effectively used. In addition, the videophone network allows children and families at home to be introduced to each other, providing mutual support and assistance. Technological visits between families with similar conditions permits families to demonstrate pulmonary care techniques and nursing procedures to each other and exchange information and experiences [15]. Tele-home health has demonstrated major cost benefits and encouraged positive patient experiences and satisfaction [16, 17].

The Everest Extreme Expedition represents perhaps the ultimate global potential outreach of telemedicine. The purpose was to provide care in a remote, extreme environment that could be applied to the home environment. The expedition permitted daily real-time high-altitude physiologic monitoring and assessment despite the hostile environment. Monitoring devices included pulse oxymetry, portable ultrasound, hand-held serum chemistry/blood gasses, electronic stethoscope, digital spirometry, digital video/imaging and photography and physiologic transport monitors. Daily linkup between Mt. Everest base camp (20 000 ft altitude) and Yale University (USA) integrated satellite, ground, and digital networks that permitted video conferencing, satellite phone conversations, and e-mail communications. The connections required only low bandwidth and used commercial off-the-shelf products and existing communications systems [18].

"If these devices could work on the mountain, their applications are limitless in the homes of patients suffering from chronic diseases such as …emphysema".

"Performance …can also be extrapolated to wider elements of global health care (*www.everestextreme99.org*)" [19].

The Present: What is the Current Evidence for the Value of Telemedicine?

In the United States, the Agency for Healthcare Research and Quality (AHRQ) serves to provide evidence-based research on issues relating to medical practices and technology assessment. The AHRQ conducted a comprehensive evaluation-based study to determine the evidence for the value of telemedicine in the Medicare (over 65) population [20]. The AHRQ considered telemedicine as the use of tele-communication technology for medical diagnosis, monitoring, and therapeutic purposes when distance separates the users. The study objective was assessment of three categories of telemedicine services that substitute face-to-face medical diagnosis and treatment in elderly patients:

1. *Store and Forward*: the collection of clinical data to store and later forward for interpretation. This technique can capture and store digital still and moving images, audio, and text. The communication is asynchronous and non-interactive with no need for patients and clinicians to be available in the same time and place. The question asked: Was this an acceptable alternative to real-time consultation?

2. *Self-Monitoring and Testing*: the monitoring of physiologic measurements, test results, images, sounds from the home/long-term care facility for post-acute and chronic care management for patients with limited mobility. The purpose was to reduce inconvenient and costly face-to-face visits. The question asked: Is it possible to provide better care through earlier detection?

3. *Clinician-Interactive Telemedicine*: real-time clinician-patient interaction that requires face-to-face visits, including on-line office visits, consultations, hospital visits, home visits, specialized examinations and procedures. The question asked: What are the cost benefits and is there physician and patient satisfaction?

The AHRQ conducted a comprehensive search for on-going programs, activities and services around the world from literature databases and Internet sites. They searched all peer-reviewed literature for efficacy and cost, and identified experts and reference lists. The AHRQ identified procedures and services supported or not supported by published studies, identified gaps in telemedicine research, and identified procedures where there was no evidence of efficacy in peer-reviewed scientific journals.

The AHRQ search reviewed 455 telemedicine programs world-wide covering 35 medical specialties and serving many diverse populations. They noted that numbers of encounters were increasing steadily but all benefits and evidence for value were equivocal and questionable. They identified only 77 articles on efficacy, of which only 9 were randomized controlled trials. The majority of programs were based at academic medical centers or hospital-based health care networks and most were providing outreach to rural locations. Their major functions were consultation or second opinion, emergency triage, specialist's visits, and tele-home health monitoring.

The AHRQ concluded that the use of telemedicine is still limited but growing and that existing programs demonstrate operational technology with potential benefits. Studies to assess efficacy and cost used inadequate methodology and were insufficient to permit definitive statements about evidence to support use.

What are the Current Trends to Consider for the Future of Health Care?

Current trends must be identified and evaluated to allow predictions. Such trends can then be used to build possible scenarios (things that might happen) of what might become the future (things we think will happen). In regard to future of health care, there are several global trends that indicate the increasing value of telemedicine.

Changing Demographics: Aging Population and Chronic Health

Many nations today are facing demands made by the increasing percentage of elderly persons. People are living longer and healthier lives. This is due in part to the advances of medicine and public health in the 20th century. However, these people are also living with long-term chronic illness and disability issues that require more healthcare and social service resources. As they advance in age, they become more of an economic burden to their families and society. They prefer, and their health would benefit, if they were able to remain at home with the support of interactive communications, monitoring, and access to health information.

In addition to the elderly, chronic diseases and disabilities have grown in significance in the general population due to growth of health issues resulting from environmental conditions, poor nutrition, and unhealthy life styles (especially due to the use of tobacco). Epidemics, especially chronic lung disease, take an enormous toll worldwide, in both human and economic terms. Nations seek ways to reduce the impact of these epidemics and to use information and communication technologies for education and health service delivery.

Health Care Finance: Long-Term Health Care Policies and Health Care Reform

Long-term care as a public policy issue has only recently been addressed. In 1990, newly re-unified Germany was one nation facing the growth of long-term care needs of an increasing elderly population. An historic meeting at the Max Planck

Institute for Social Science Research brought together an interdisciplinary group of social and political scientists, economists, and health experts from many nations to determine how other countries adapted to the chronic health needs of their aging populations [21]. These policy experts sought innovative approaches to organize and finance health care delivery. Home care facilitates chronic care in many nations. Being connected at home to health information with interactive monitoring and communications could support many more people with long-term chronic health needs.

In 2001, an interactive television program in the United States dramatized the growing impact of long-term health issues in the lives of many families and communities [22]. It was noted that 125 million Americans lived with at least one chronic health problem and this was expected to grow to 157 million in the next 20 years. Furthermore, these people received care directly by "informal caregivers" and/or economic support from one in four Americans (either family members or friends), the majority of whom were working mothers caring for both their parents and their own children. The economic burden of the out-of-pocket expenses for the support of these elderly persons was estimated to be $ 500 billion annually and total direct costs were expected to reach $ 1 trillion (about 80% of total health care spending) [22]. This burden was due, in part, to the lack of interest in long-term care because of an inadequate comprehensive long-term health care policy.

Every nation faces the challenge to meet the increasing burden of growing health care costs. As nations evaluate possible options, they realize that long-term care is a major cost issue. The current approaches to chronic disease and disabilities are fragmented and restrictive. Policies include competitive bidding for the least-expensive alternatives and coding practices that limit use of life-sustaining and cost-saving medical equipment and communication technologies. Policies of the past have not adapted to current chronic health needs or fostered changes in health care delivery that would improve the lives of patients and families. More costly facility-based care is often the only option when less expensive home and alternative community settings would be preferable and more health promoting. Long-term care is now a subject for inclusion in many nations' global health reform debates.

*Health Care Organization: Disease Management Protocols
and Community Health Networks*

When chronic health conditions are only managed intermittently for acute crises and major complications, the economic burden to patients, their families and society is enormous. Disease management programs have come from the need to reduce cost, improve quality and determine optimal health outcomes. These evidence-based programs are part of a trend to create an integrated, collaborative team approach. The disease management concept represents a paradigm shift away from episodic to long-term care strategies [23]. Disease management protocols are being used to facilitate care by connecting multiple care sites (facility and community settings), by improving health care resource utilization and integrating information and communication with electronic medical records and administrative management.

The multidisciplinary approach with a broad range of medical expertise across the continuum of care (acute, sub-acute, and chronic) is fundamental to the success of disease management. The team required consists of professionals including physicians, nurses, pharmacists, home care, clinical researchers, data analysts, quality control specialists, actuarial experts and case managers, among others. This comprehensive approach to long-term care has been recently promoted by the US Department of Health and Human Services (HHS) Center for Medicare and Medicaid Services (CMS) by supporting Chronic Care Improvement Organizations (CCIP) [24, 25].

Many of the factors causing chronic health problems are due to social, economic, cultural, environmental and political issues. There is an increasing trend to view chronic illness as a global health challenge that requires the integration of medical practice and public health. Community Health Networks are bringing together public, private, and voluntary sectors to foster cooperation and collaboration at the community level. For example, the Chicago Asthma Consortium (CAC) has a decade of experience uniting the community to curb the epidemic of asthma in ways that can only be accomplished collectively. The CAC is a knowledge community involved in gathering data, disseminating information, and fostering communication [26].

Consumer Preferences: Seeking Knowledge for Self-Care

Patients and families demand more involvement in self-management of their long-term health needs. This is an evolution of the "self-help" movement for family-centered, family-directed health care. More people have already become accustomed to using modern means of communication (cellular, mobile, satellite, computer) in their everyday lives. They expect and seek improved access to information to make all decisions, especially related to health care, which is the number one topic of interest and reason they use the Internet [27]. People join global knowledge communities to learn more about how to manage their health and communicate with their physicians. Many elderly people are becoming capable of using the Internet (the "wired-retired") [27]. They are motivated to do so to keep in contact with family members and to seek information to facilitate their lives.

The power of information for chronic health management was recognized over a quarter of century ago. Providing prescribed information as a medical service is known as "information therapy". Information therapy means "the right information to the right person at the right time" (time of decision/action) [5]. More recently, a demonstration of providing information to the community has become a means of chronic disease management for people experiencing disparities in health care. In Philadelphia, Community Health Information Centers (CHIC) fill in the physician-information prescription which provides necessary health education for self-management and enhances compliance with the pharmaceutical prescription [6].

Technological Advances: Tools that Facilitate Health Care Delivery and Management

Over the last decade, advances in computerized information management, mobile communication technologies, and portable medical devices have converged, facilitating connectivity and information exchange. This has permitted the growth of the practice of telemedicine for monitoring chronic health conditions in communities especially in remote and rural regions when encouraged by health care policy and finance. Telehealth services are used to integrate clinical information and administrative data to facilitate service delivery as well as outcome evaluation. In this regard, there has been a convergence of clinical support based on disease management protocols to manage care, improve quality and reduce costs. Home care can now provide continuous monitoring of situations for early detection of health concerns, to identify emergencies, to assure compliance with treatment plans, and to maintain surveillance that can reduce more expensive direct travel to the home. The medical devices as well as communication technology are simple and relatively inexpensive as are the services that provide them. As already noted, studies have revealed satisfaction with telehealth visits by providers as well as patients and families.

Physician Practice Changes: Integrating Information into Clinical Management

The practice of medicine demands access to and appropriate use of information. Physicians (especially younger ones who grew up using computers and the Internet) rely on electronic information to update their own knowledge and to become current with the latest medical knowledge and evidence-based practice guidelines. Physicians also use information technology to supplement education of their patients for their self-management. Pagers have been replaced by mobile/cellular technology making interactive communication easier. In addition, physicians will communicate by e-mail when appropriate expectations and disclosures have been defined. Using computers and hand-held personal devices facilitates physician communication and makes it easier to obtain patient and administrative data and to integrate the care of patients across the care continuum and in alternative care settings in electronic medical records. Physicians use telemedicine to monitor patient conditions between communications, identify urgent changes/trends in health conditions requiring attention, and facilitate patient compliance with disease management protocols.

The Vision: A Preferred Scenario for the Future

"If we could first know where we are, and whither we are tending, we could better judge what to do and how to do it." (Abraham Lincoln)

Why should we consider "the future"? Although we cannot know the future for certain, we can, by what we do, or do not do, help determine our future. For this reason we need to monitor current trends (what is happening now) to construct possible future scenarios (what might happen) and chose our preferred scenario (what we want to happen). We can plan a strategic direction, we can make choices, determine priorities, and direct our course of action, and we and must do this as individuals, organizations, and as diverse communities working together.

There are multiple scenarios that could be constructed based on current trends that involve telemedicine. They reflect health care delivery changes and the degree/rapidity of that change. The following scenarios reflect the future of health care in general in the author's country (the USA, which has a market approach with many restrictive regulations). There are, however, global implications. The conclusions from the 1990 Max Planck conference noted that a nation's "finance system" has less impact than cultural difference between countries. What is important is that funding is provided to encourage innovation and change, and that change occurs in the appropriate cultural context [21].

Current Health Care Delivery: Remains Unchanged

There will be increased cut-throat competition among service and equipment providers. A growing number of uninsured employed people will be denied access to care. More expensive institutional care will be the limited option requiring more travel time (less worker productivity), and cost to employers, patients and families. Patients will gravitate to alternative care providers and delivery models that provide on-line services. Care will be poorly coordinated with poor communication.

Current Health Care Delivery: Incremental Change

There will be more collaborative care arrangements integrating services from multiple providers who have increasing bargaining influence in the market and with public agencies. New health care finance models will feature greater patient responsibility and control. Community-based, integrated care settings will be established which provide tele-care and tele-consultation to supplement intermittent visits (changing care from episodic acute interventions to continuous health management). These models will integrate complementary/alternative medicine and public health with traditional medical practices.

Current Health Care Delivery: Radical Change

The office of the future will integrate electronic medical data and communications at every point of service. There will be convenient care at multiple sites from professionals and non-professional assistants. There will be universal access to medical records with appropriate protection of patient privacy (e-files). Digital sensors and video technology will permit remote monitoring with feedback loop modifications. Telehealth will permit self-care at home with robotic assistants supplementing informal family care providers, interactive e-mail communication, and web-based education. There will be changes in living conditions to promote healthier living styles that will make health care more appropriate by distance management, rather than by travel to health care centers.

Global Health Vision for Telemedicine and e-Health

The following vision-directed preferred scenario will be possible if people work together toward a mutually desired future. Adapting a shared vision mobilizes, energizes, encourages and motivates all persons concerned. A vision facilitates team synergy and interdependency... and people might just get what they want!

Patient-Physician Partnering: Collaboration, Communication and Coordination

With access to interactive tele-communication and knowledge-based services, patients and families will become educated and involved in chronic disease self-management. They will be more informed to understand and communicate with their physicians and other health providers. They will accept more responsibility and be more compliant in the health management plan which they will accept since they had a role in its development.

Chronic Disease Management: Practice Guidelines and Evidence-Based Protocols

Health care services and medical resource utilization will be guided by outcome-driven evidence-based clinical protocols. These protocols will be developed with the input of all constituents that have a stake in improving patient safety in the home, enhancing quality of life, and managing costs within reasonable and defined limitations. Such protocols will be integrated by informatics/communications systems that will provide information when and where it is needed to make decisions, take actions, and modify existing treatment plans. These systems will be patient/family centric and involve case managers with clinical and management expertise.

Long-Term Care Continuous Monitoring and Improvement

With tele-monitoring, communication, and consultation possible in the home and other community settings, care will become continuous and focused on health promotion despite the chronic nature of the diseases or disabilities. Patients, physicians, and providers will have all-year round access to information and communication. Management decisions and patient compliance with plans will be integrated with data trend analysis to determine medically necessary changes. Patients can reach their doctors, explain their current health situation and needs; physicians can respond with guidance and determine optimal moments for patient/family education. Pooled data can be analyzed for outcomes to determine validity of individual management plans, guidelines in general and for improvement by integration of clinical care and health service quality/cost management.

Overcoming Health Care Disparities due to Distance, Time, Access, and Cost

Chronic disease management will be facilitated by physician generalists and other health professionals (nurses, nurse practitioners, social workers, allied health professionals, case managers) with enhanced access to medical and surgical specialists. Specialty health care delivery at facility-based medical centers and/or from the concentration of specialty services located in urban and suburban areas will be extended to rural and remote areas. Professional and patient/family access to specialist's knowledge, expertise, consultation and management will be facilitated by interactive telecommunication of data, text, audio, video and images. Data will be collected and outcome analyzed for population-based health focusing on chronic conditions where greater impact can be made by a global health (integrated public health and medical practice) approach.

A Call for Descriptive Experience and for Outcome-Based Evaluation Research

Chronic lung disease has become a prominent and growing cause of morbidity and mortality world-wide. Not only patients and families, but also society, suffers a great deal due to the economic costs of lost worker productivity and the health care and social services required. Whatever can be done to improve quality of health and life and maintain such patients at home with their families will have great impact on managed care and global health finances.

Telehealth (telemedicine and e-health) has potential to allow the continuous monitoring of patient status in the home, educating patients and families for self-management, and assuring compliance with medical plans. Intermittent acute care can be transformed into long-term health management of chronic conditions. Telecommunication (especially by e-mail) can provide earlier, more regular communication between patients and physicians and foster a collaborative partnership. Integrating public health and disease management protocols can assure a more global approach to chronic illness and potentially improve health outcomes. Using electronic medical records and information systems to manage the logistics and resources of health care delivery can provide operational efficiencies with significantly improved economic outcomes.

The 2001 AHRQ evaluated modalities of telemedicine in clinical management of elderly patients and provides a "call to action". We can achieve a desired future scenario with benefits to all sectors of society. However, due to the limitations of resources for health and social services, it is mandatory that we have rigorous descriptions and analyses of experiences that can document that they have made a difference. The remainder of this book describes such an experience with the clinical use and management of long-term oxygen in the home for chronic respiratory insufficiency. This experience is important for people around the world who are interested in the future of health care from many perspectives. This is the first and essential step toward the health service research required for planning an evaluation-driven system.

References

1. Reid J (1996) Telemedicine primer. Understanding the issues. Innovative medical Communications. Topeka, Kansas (Available at: 1-800-409-9706)
2. American Academy of Family Physicians (2005) Telemedicine. Telehealth Discussion Paper. www.aafp.org/x17523.xml Accessed April 15, 2005
3. Washington State Board of Health (1997) Telemedicine: A Report to the Legislature
4. National Academy of Sciences, Institute of Medicine (1995) Telemedicine: A Guide to Assessing Telecommunication in Healthcare. National Academy Press, Washington, DC
5. Kemper DW, Mettler M (2002) Information Therapy: Prescribed Information as a Reimbursable Medical Service. Center for Information Therapy (Healthwise, Boise, ID)
6. College of Physicians of Philadelphia. Community Health Information Centers www.collphyphil.org/chic.html; www.phillyhealthinfo.org Accessed April 15, 2005
7. Bynum A, Hopkins D, Thomas A, Copeland N, Irwin C (2001) The effect of telepharmacy counseling on meter-dose inhaler techniques among adolescents with asthma in rural Arkansas. Telemed J E Health 7(3):207-217
8. Kristo DA, Eliasson AH, Poropatich RK, Netzer CM, Bradley JP, Louke DI, Netzer NC (2001) Telemedicine in the sleep laboratory. Feasibility and economic advantages of polysomnography transferred on-line. Telemed J E Health 7(3):219-224

9. Hnatiuk OW (2001) Interpretation of adult spirometry using telemedicine. Telemed J E Health 7(2):149
10. Meyer MA, Ryan P (2001) The Veteran's Administration Care Management System: The marriage of care coordination and technology in the home – matching patient population with technologies. Telemed J E Health 7(2):135-136
11. Vogel DC (2001) Monitor health status and deliver health education in the home. Telemed J E Health 7(2):151
12. Agha A, Schapira RM (2001) Telemedicine for the delivery of pulmonary outpatient care in a rural site: a cost analysis. Telemed J E Health 7(2):149
13. US Army Surgeon General Policy (2005) Use of Army Knowledge Online Email in Support of Electronic Telehealth Medical Consultation by Deployed Providers: OSTG/MEDCOM Policy Memo 05-004, 17 March
14. Miyasaka K, Suzuki Y, Sakai H, Kondo Y (1997) Interactive communication in high-technology home care: videophones for pediatric ventilatory care. Pediatrics 99:1e-6e
15. Adachi T, Miyasaka K (1996) A case study of interactive communication by videophone between parents with handicapped children. Tohuko Psychologica Folia 55:34-38
16. Dansky KHP, Palmer L, Shea D, Bowles KH (2001) Cost analysis of tele-homecare. Telemed J E Health 7(3):225-232
17. Demeris G, Speedie SM, Finkelstein S (2001) Change of patients' perceptions of tele-homecare. Telemed J E Health 7(3):241-248
18. Angood PB, Satava R, Doarn C, Morrell R, E3 Group (2000) Medicine at the top of the world. The 1998 and 1999 Everest Extreme Expedition. Telemed J E Health 6(3):315-325
19. Telemedicine proves its mettle on Mt. Everest (1999) Yale Medicine 33(3):5-6
20. Hersh WR, Wallace JA, Patterson RK, Shapiro SE, Kraemer DF, Eilers GM, Chan BKS, Greenlkick MR, Helfand M (2001) Telemedicine for the Medicare Population. Evidence Report/Technology Assessment #24. Agency for Healthcare Research and Quality. AHRQ Publication No. 01-E012. Rockville, MD, July 2001
21. Hollingsworth JR, Hollingsworth EJ (1994) Care of the chronically and severely ill: comparative social policies. New York: Aldene de Gruyter, (Reports from a 1990 Conference at the Max Planck Institut for Social Policy Research, Cologne, Germany)
22. Who Cares: Chronic Illness in America. Fred Friendly Seminar www.pbs.org/fredfriendly/whocares/about_the_program/about_the_program.html Accessed April 15, 2005
23. Lehmann C, Giacini JM (2004) Tele-health and disease management. The Remington Report 12(4):14-18
24. Schwartz RM (2004) News Reports from Washington. New Chronic Care Program Noted. The Remington Report 12(4):36-38
25. Remington L (2004) CMS (Centers for Medicare and Medicaid Services) demonstrations projects under the Medicare Prescription Drug Improvement and Modernization Act. The Remington Report 12(4):20-22
26. www.chicagoasthma.org Accessed April 15, 2004
27. Conversations with Dr. Koop. www.chestnet.org/CHEST/past/koop/ Accessed April 15, 2004

Home Long-Term Oxygen Treatment (H-LTOT): Why, Where, and How

R.W. Dal Negro

The story of long-term oxygen treatment (LTOT) begins in 1774, with the discovery of oxygen by Joseph Priestley, and his description of the element as having a "peculiarly salutary effect to the lungs in certain morbid cases". Priestley's suggestions were put into practice a couple of decades later by Dr. Thomas Beddoes who used oxygen as a therapeutic agent in clinics and published his own experiences in 1798.

Since that period, a huge amount of data has become available concerning the physiological and patho-physiological mechanisms of oxygen uptake, oxygen delivery, and the effects of oxygen on metabolism in different human tissues.

The knowledge that 30 molecules of adenosine tri-phosphate (such as high energy ATP) can be generated from each molecule of glucose in the presence of oxygen, as opposed to only 3 ATP molecules and lactic acid in its absence, further emphasized oxygen's therapeutic potential.

Factors influencing both oxygen uptake and delivery were investigated extensively in the last century from morphological, physiological, and biological points of view, with particular emphasis on the consequences of hypoxemia. Respiratory patients are faced with a range of conditions, including parenchymal destruction, changes in lung structures leading to subsequent reduction in gas diffusion, alveolar hypo-ventilation (when hypoxemia combines with hypercapnia), the ventilation-to-perfusion mis-match (when the under-ventilation of a number of alveoli cannot be compensated by the over-ventilation of other groups of alveoli due to the sigmoid shape of the oxygen-hemoglobin dissociation curve), alterations in blood perfusion and changes in the hemoglobin affinity to oxygen. Investigation of these conditions allowed clarification of the effects of hypoxemia in humans, and definition of the most appropriate strategies for hypoxemia correction.

Oxygen supplementation has become an irreplaceable therapeutic weapon in patients with various respiratory diseases. In particular, in the second half of the last century, oxygen supplementation was suggested as a particularly promising therapeutic option for the treatment of chronic respiratory conditions, such as severe chronic obstructive pulmonary disease (COPD), chronic respiratory (or cardio-respiratory) failure, lung fibrosis, kyphoscoliosis and other thoracic deformities, chronic cor pulmonale, and severe respiratory sleep disorders.

These patients have severe and persistent hypoxemia, need daily oxygen treatments and their basal clinical condition undergoes severe exacerbations (an average of 3-4 times per year) due to diverse causes (infectious or inflammatory), or worsening of concomitant conditions which precipitate hypoxemia.

Moreover, in the presence of fixed airway obstruction, chronic hypoxemia may occur even during light exercise and can also occur in patients who prove normoxic at rest. Life threatening levels of hypoxemia are frequent during acute exacerbations of COPD, when hypercapnia and respiratory acidosis can combine. It is mainly these patients that are treated with LTOT, prescribed to reduce or minimize the dangerous effects of severe hypoxemia, which is frequently associated with sleep disorders and pulmonary hypertension.

In general terms, respiratory failure can be defined as the presence of hypoxemia (such as PaO_2 <60 mmHg at rest, breathing ambient air at sea level) due to respiratory causes. Hypoxemia can combine with normocapnia (type 1 respiratory failure), or with hypercapnia (type 2 respiratory failure). The latter condition presents the greatest risk to the patient's life and to his clinical management. In these conditions the appropriate level of oxygen delivered and maximal CO_2 toleration levels should be precisely assessed before determining the relevant long-term therapeutic strategy.

In the past, patient survival was used as the bench-mark for judging the success of the treatment. However, in recent years other factors, in particular quality of life, have been regarded as crucial considerations for assessing different long-term therapeutic strategies.

The new era in LTOT started when it was established that home LTOT (H-LTOT) could improve survival in subjects suffering from severe hypoxemia due to COPD [1-3]. The beneficial effects of H-LTOT were assessed for the first time by two pivotal long-term studies carried out in the mid-Seventies and early Eighties. These two controlled clinical studies definitively demonstrated that LTOT is the only therapeutic option able *per se* to prolong the life of subjects suffering from type 2 chronic respiratory failure due to severe COPD and emphysema, characterized by fixed airway obstruction and a PaO_2 <55 mmHg (with the patients conscious and breathing air) [2, 3]. In particular, these studies proved that only about 30% of patients survive for three years without oxygen supplementation, that daily 12-15 hour oxygen administration leads to a significant improvement in survival rates, and that the best survival is obtained following more than 19 hours of oxygen administration within a period of 24 hours (Fig. 1). Moreover, LTOT was also proven to partially reverse pulmonary hypertension [3, 4].

A few years later, re-analysis of the Nocturnal Oxygen Therapy Trial (NOTT) also proved that the best survival was seen in those subjects who showed a significant, if small, decrease in basal pulmonary hypertension during LTOT [5]. Interestingly, patients with type 2 chronic respiratory failure on LTOT also showed a significant reduction in secondary polycythemia, a factor leading to a significant improvement in quality of life [6, 7].

Even though these pivotal controlled studies confirmed the therapeutic value of LTOT for the first time, they also proved that, depending on the chronic respiratory patient's original lung function profile, LTOT can lead to different clinical outcomes. In fact, oxygen therapy does not benefit all patients and thus patients should be carefully investigated before being included in a LTOT program, particularly when they are entirely home-managed.

Obviously, criteria for selecting patients is the true crucial point for the optimiza-

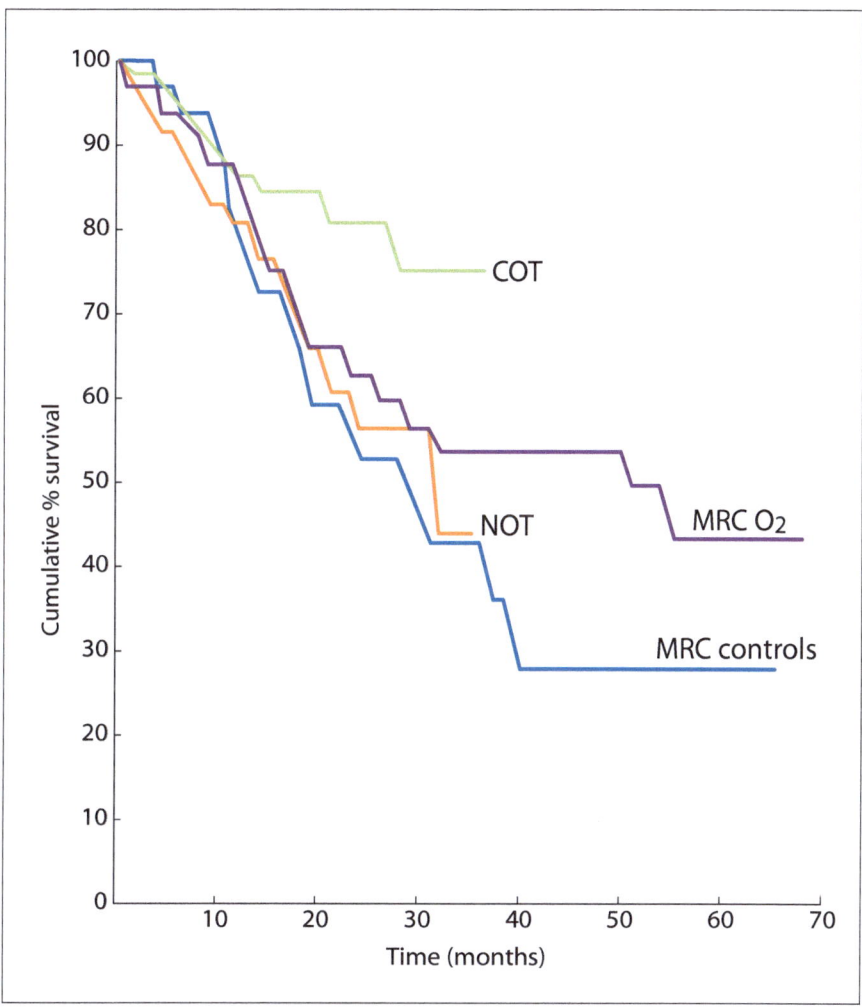

Fig. 1. Survival with LTOT in different groups of patients. MRC controls did not receive oxygen; NOT and MRC O$_2$ received oxygen for 12 and 15 hours/day, respectively; COT subjects received oxygen for more than 19 hours/day (Modified from [3])

tion of both therapeutic efficacy and effectiveness of LTOT. The selection criteria also significantly impact on the success of LTOT, in both social and economic terms.

Originally, a high arterial PCO$_2$ and an elevated erythrocyte mass appeared to be the best indicators of patients who would benefit most from LTOT in terms of long-term survival; other patients who benefited showed a 5 mmHg decrease in arterial pulmonary pressure following administration of 28% oxygen for 24 hours [2, 8]. On the contrary, excessive ventilation upon exercise was suggested as a predictor of poor survival in these patients; in particular, patients with a ratio of minute ventilation/CO$_2$ output of more than 31 were likely to die in three years, independent of oxygen administration [8].

In the first half of the Eighties, oxygen therapy was mainly recommended to

Table 1. Most frequent causes of chronic respiratory failure needing LTOT (1986, internal data; n=111)

COPD	68.4%
Kyphoscoliosis	10.8%
Lung fibrosis	6.3%
Pulmonary embolism	5.4%
Pneumoconiosis	5.4%
Lung cancer	2.7%
Other	1.0%

patients suffering from severe COPD (major conditions leading to recommendation of LTOT over twenty years are reported in Table 1). Stable COPD patients with chronic and appropriate pharmacological treatment, who show a PaO_2 persistently <55 mmHg while breathing ambient air for at least 20 minutes and confirmed by two arterial blood samples three weeks apart were considered suitable for LTOT. Further criteria were a PaO_2 of 55-59 mmHg when combined with cor pulmonale, or a hematocrit greater than 55%. In these conditions, oxygen saturation was increased by continuous oxygen flow and maintained in the range 88-94% during LTOT [2, 3].

LTOT was also supposed to benefit restrictive patients, or patients suffering from other chronic respiratory and/or cardio-respiratory diseases even though in these cases LTOT has less clinical impact in both short and long-term programs (see chapter 6).

Particular attention was also paid to subjects suffering from severe hypoxemia during REM sleep, and in whom oxygen administration led to the correction of their sleep desaturation episodes. In these conditions, oxygen supplementation can actually cause a significant decrease in arterial pulmonary pressure, which normally increases during REM sleep.

LTOT should be carefully considered and managed when CO_2 retention is present because this might be aggravated by oxygen administration; in these cases the combined use of continuous positive airway pressure (C-PAP) has long proven crucial [9].

In general terms, long-term controlled oxygen therapy was soon regarded as an essential therapeutic option, and gained an established position in the care of selected respiratory subjects with persistent hypoxemia in both chronic conditions and during acute exacerbations of respiratory dysfunctions.

Results of the first studies highlighted immediately that improved survival, reduced hospitalization, improved exercise tolerance, and better quality of life were the most relevant factors to monitor in order to assess the true efficacy and effectiveness of LTOT in long-term prospective studies. In particular, these studies focused on severe COPD patients, whose chronic respiratory and general conditions were usually as debilitating as those of some cancer sufferers. Following the NOTT and the MRC studies [2, 3], LTOT was used in both Europe and the US according to different protocols and territorial strategies, and H-LTOT started in several countries according to models established by their health care organizations. In the UK in 1991, the rate of LTOT prescription was 16/100 000 inhabitants [10].

France played a pioneering role in this field because it very quickly adopted LTOT strategies [11]. By 1975 a sample of more than 500 subjects had been already investigated and consistent data on global outcomes was garnered from a large population of patients suffering from chronic respiratory failure undergoing LTOT. Management of the patients was overseen by regional associations, which were also created in France at that time, grouped in a National Association (ANTADIR, *Association Nationale pour le Traitment à Domicile de l'Insuffisance Respiratoire Chronique*); a very efficient network for patient care has been built up since the end of the Seventies. Information concerning more than 8000 patients was available a few years later, thus significantly improving the basic know-how of H-LTOT management. The Ministry of Health and the *Caisse Nationale d'Assurance Maladie* supported a national study which included 200 hospitals, more than 120 insurance companies and more than 600 patients from several chest departments. In 1979, 50 000 French patients were suffering from chronic respiratory failure, of whom 11 000 (22%) had some domiciliary respiratory assistance (7000 had oxygen only for variable periods over 24 hours, and 1000 were mechanically ventilated). Patient follow-up was carried out by local associations and sometimes by hospital departments, but many patients remained uncontrolled due to the absence of any association in their region. For this reason, the LTOT results were variable, proving that local organization and economic situation are critical aspects which need to be taken into account. A decade later, local and national associations had evolved, with more structure and available full-time medical staff, allowing the problems associated with LTOT to be faced in a much more organized and pragmatic way. Currently in France, each patient that needs home support for chronic respiratory problems is registered by ANTADIR and by local associations, greatly facilitating both national investigations and education programs, and stimulating research.

Another important survey of the living conditions of severe chronic respiratory patients treated at home by LTOT or assisted ventilation was carried out in 1990. Several regional associations and more than 13 000 subjects were surveyed by questionnaire in order to determine their self-sufficiency, their daily life, and their handling of equipment at home. The patients' behavioural profiles were established and the data collected was of great utility in planning further educational studies oriented to the amelioration of patient compliance to H-LTOT programs [12].

Other countries contributed to LTOT development. The National Registry of Sweden, begun in the late Eighties, revealed that 70% of patients in LTOT were COPD patients [13]. In the USA, the problems of LTOT and of mechanical ventilation at home have been approached differently. There is no mechanism of accountability to ensure that homecare prescription and delivery are adequate, nor is there reimbursement for services, educational programs for the patients or their families, communication or documentation of information, or technological improvement. Furthermore, patient safety and cost-saving are not part of a regionalized

Table 2. The role of patient compliance on clinical outcomes. Highly compliant patients had significantly lower exacerbations and hospital admissions both in spring/summer and in autumn/winter periods. A score > or <1 was considered discriminant (1986, internal data)

	Compliance			
	High level score =1.2 (n=24)		Low level score= 0.45 (n=19)	
	Hospital admissions (%)	Exacerbations (%)	Hospital admissions (%)	Exacerbations (%)
Spring/summer	8.3	12.5	44.4*	58.9*
Autumn/winter	20.8	33.3	66.7*	88.9*

*p<0.05 (Wilcoxon test between groups)

association model of intervention oriented to the proper attention of cost-containment and quality-assurance.

In Japan, a national register of patients treated in a LTOT regimen started in 1986 and by 1993 more than 32 000 patients were included. The register documents survival rates and outcomes according to patient gender, regardless of the cause of their respiratory failure [14].

The absolute value of continuous LTOT in the management of chronic respiratory failure was further emphasized in different studies carried out during the last decade, with repeated confirmations of the indications and selection criteria for patients to be included in LTOT programs [15]. It was also confirmed that oxygen should be used for at least 15 hours per day; a shorter period of oxygen administration is regarded as an insufficient and ineffective strategy in terms of increasing life expectancy and improving pulmonary hypertension.

Once the administration of oxygen for many hours per day is accepted, the role of patient compliance and adherence to the program becomes another crucial and critical point (Table 2), with the role of the family and care-givers absolutely relevant in obtaining the benefits of home therapeutic protocols.

The development and implementation of portable devices for LTOT has rapidly facilitated daily adherence and length of oxygen treatment, thus improving patient quality of life by significantly lowering the level of disability. The advances have enabled an increase in time spent in domestic activities and leisure, as well as the number of hours spent outside the patient's home. Recently, new evidence suggested that a decisive impact on perceived quality of life of mobile LTOT patients depends on the patient's equipment selection. In fact, those patients on liquid oxygen show an improved quality of life compared to subjects administered oxygen via concentrator or gas cylinder [16].

One parameter of LTOT that is challenging to establish is the way in which oxygen should be administered; that is, at rest, during sleep or during exercise. An international survey was carried out via questionnaire in order to determine how specialists in several different countries prescribe oxygen [17]. The vast majority of respondents tended to customize the oxygen prescription starting from information collected at rest, but the approach to night prescription was quite diverse. While spe-

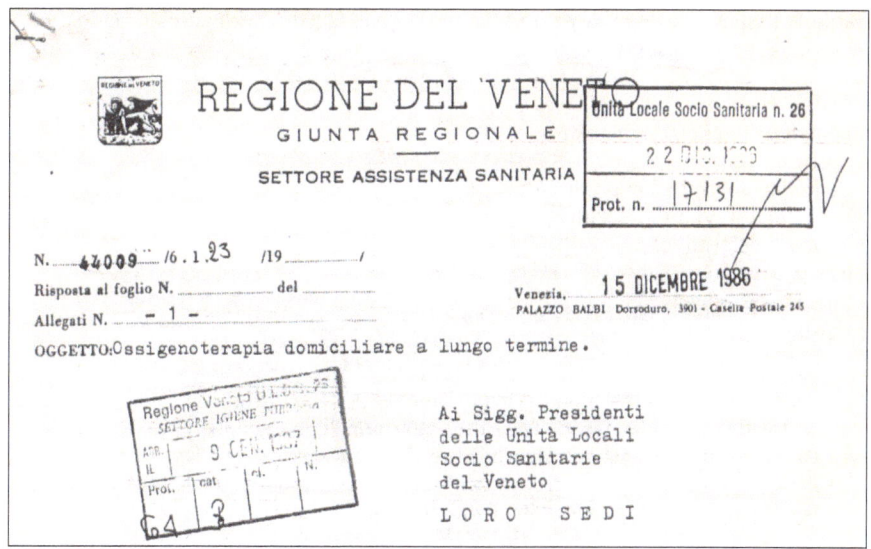

Fig. 2. The first institutional regulatory document concerning LTOT in Italy was issued in 1986 by the Department for Public Health and Social Affairs of the *Regione Veneto*

cialists in Canada and in the USA usually increase the resting oxygen flow only during sleep, in Spain the oxygen resting flow is usually maintained during sleep; while in France, the Netherlands and Italy the night-time oxygen prescription is assessed much more frequently. Substantial international differences were also seen in terms of criteria for individualizing oxygen prescription during exercise [17].

Another challenging aspect affecting LTOT is the absence of standardized assessment protocols to compare outcomes among patients receiving H-LTOT. This particular problem is further magnified because, as described in the UK, H-LTOT is frequently prescribed and provided by general practitioners, with the reasons for the initial prescription often obscure, and their decision criteria often outside the prescribing guidelines [18]. In Scotland, even though LTOT has been prescribed only by respiratory specialists since 1989, compliance to LTOT ranges widely and is similar to that observed in other studies carried out in countries where general practitioners can prescribe this treatment [19].

H-LTOT was accepted with great favour in Italy in the Eighties and a few groups immediately started to investigate different aspects of this new therapeutic approach to severe chronic hypoxemic patients. The attention of Italian specialists at that time was initially focused on the true effectiveness of LTOT, together with the effectiveness of the different devices for oxygen delivery and patient compliance.

While there was no national regulation for managing LTOT, the first Italian institutional regulatory document concerning LTOT was issued by the Department for Public Health of the *Regione Veneto* in 1986 (doc. no. 44009/6.1.23, December 15th, 1986) (Fig. 2). This document reported the diseases to be treated by LTOT, along with absolute and additional criteria for selecting, including and excluding LTOT patients (Table 3). Also included were the operational procedures to follow to manage H-LTOT patients effectively, while maintaining operational

Table 3. Respiratory diseases where LTOT is allowed, together with absolute and additive selection criteria for LTOT

- COPD
- Lung fibrosis and granulomatosis
- Cystic fibrosis
- Central hypoventilation syndromes
- Neurological syndromes with hypoventilation
- Thoracic deformities
- Chronic cor pulmonale
- Pneumonectomy
- Cardio-respiratory failure

   Absolute criteria
   - Persistent (at least two months) hypoxemia (PaO_2 <55 mmHg), unresponsive to regular treatments, as assessed in two different arterial blood samples (3 weeks apart)
   - PaO_2 improvement >60 mmHg while breathing oxygen
   - $PaCO_2$ not increasing dangerously while breathing oxygen
   - Persistent hypoxemia concomitant with $PaCO_2$ <55 mmHg

   Additive criteria
   - Occurrence of hypoxemic (or desaturation) episodes during sleep even though the patient is normoxemic when awake
   - PaO_2 between 56-65 mmHg in the presence of documented PaO_2 <60 mmHg during exercise (40 watts)
   - Ischemic heart disease
   - Pulmonary hypertension
   - Hematocrit value >55 %

contacts with general practitioners. Moreover, the document also stated that LTOT and the corresponding health arrangements had to be delivered free of charge only to those patients who fitted the selection criteria mentioned above. Oxygen was delivered from cylinders as compressed gas, from concentrators, or stored in big cylinders as liquid oxygen, and economizer devices were also considered.

Initially, concentrators were preferred for home LTOT, but problems of higher cost and environmental noise, and of lower oxygen quality, switched the interest of Italian specialists to liquid oxygen in the following years, which had the concomitant advantage of improving patient quality of life.

Despite the improved survival rates, the long-term need for oxygen administration for more than 15-18 hours per day resulted in some patients obstinantly refusing LTOT. This was considered to be mainly due to the patient's refusal to demonstrate his own disability to relatives and friends in day-to-day life. In that initial period, small groups of strictly selected patients were managed at home with the aid of volunteer care givers.

Although LTOT was regarded as a "cost-saving" option, it was actually rather costly, considering that the social and economic costs depended on the prevalence of LTOT needs within the different territories and on the cost of educating patients and their families who were included in the therapeutic program at home. In 1988, our specialist group was asked by the Department for Public Health and Social Affairs of the Regione Veneto for a triennial epidemiological investigation in order

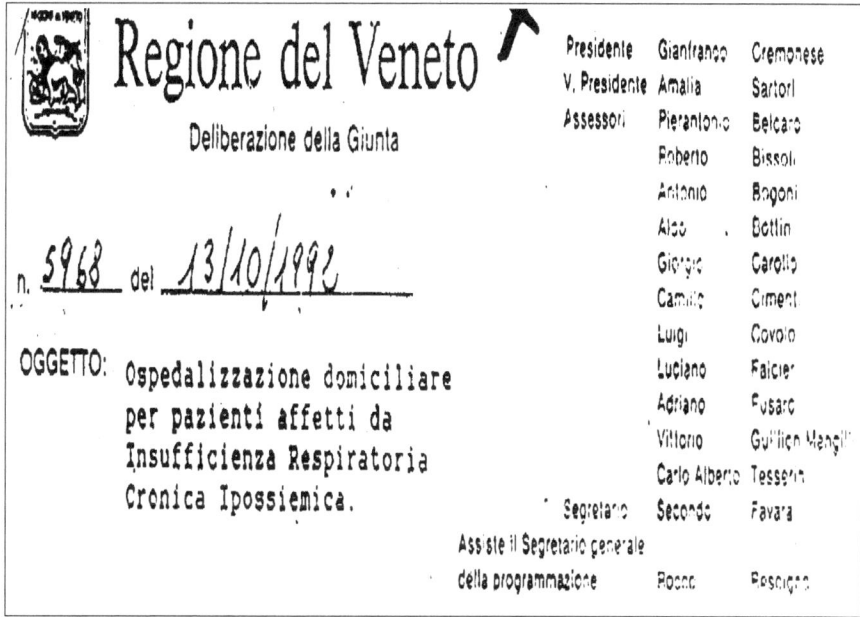

Fig. 3. The regulatory document concerning the "domiciliary hospitalization" for patients suffering from chronic respiratory failure was issued in 1992 by the department for Public Health and Social Affairs of the *Regione Veneto*

to assess the regional prevalence of LTOT within an area of 4.5 million inhabitants, and consequently to plan the investment of economic resources. This pioneer investigation was officially supported by the Regione Veneto (research no. 182/03.88) and represented the first Italian study on this topic. The 3-year study was carried out from 1988 to 1990, with a LTOT prevalence of 78/100 000 inhabitants (general population). As these results have been checked and confirmed several times in the same territories in the following fifteen years, the number is assumed to be representative of the true prevalence of LTOT in Italy.

On this basis, the Department for Public Health and Social Affairs updated the inclusion/exclusion criteria for LTOT, and a further official document stating the beginning of the "domiciliary hospitalization" for selected patients needing LTOT and/or home mechanical ventilation was issued in 1992 (Fig. 3). This document was very innovative: it ruled that patients needing LTOT would be managed at home with the same rights and facilities, both in terms of medical and nursing support, and of diagnostic and therapeutic options, as those admitted into hospital departments. The goal of the document was to reduce the number of hospital admissions for these patients and to substantially reduce the huge amount of related direct health costs, while maintaining or improving the effects of previous therapeutic treatments.

Patients and their families happily accepted this innovative opportunity, even though it meant that their specific education and training had to be urgently improved. A teaching program run by volunteers (doctors, nurses and skilled caregivers) was quickly organized to help inexperienced patients.

Table 4A, 4B. PaO_2 trend (mean values; SD; min., and max. values) assessed during an 18-month survey of patients with chronic respiratory failure who agreed (A, n=34), and who did not agree (B, controls, n=16) to the LTOT protocol at home. The increase in PaO_2 was statistically significant over the 540 days only in compliant patients

A	Bsln	90	180	360	540	Days
Mean	53.3	60.9	61.2*	63.2**	67.3**	
SD	5.7	7.6	10.1	9.2	5.2	
Min.	40.1	44.1	46.2	47.7	59.9	
Max.	60.1	69.1	66.5	69.8	71.8	

B	Bsln	90	180	360	540	Days
Mean	56.9	56.1	51.0	52.9	52.6	
SD	7.7	7.2	6.6	5.0	6.1	
Min.	46.6	51.5	49.2	51.3	52.1	
Max.	65.6	66.5	61.7	60.9	61.2	

* $p<0.05$; ** $p<0.01$ (Anova)

Table 5A, 5B. $PaCO_2$ trend (mean values; SD; min., and max. values) assessed during an 18-month survey of patients with chronic respiratory failure who agreed (A, n=34), and who did not agree (B, controls, n=16) to the LTOT protocol at home. Compared to non-compliant, only compliant patients showed $PaCO_2$ decrease, although the changes did not reach statistical significance

A	Bsln	90	180	360	540	Days
Mean	47.9	44.8	44.7	45.1	46.1	
SD	8.1	7.2	7.3	5.8	6.6	
Min.	33.5	31.9	37.0	37.1	33.4	
Max.	67.0	56.9	65.7	58.7	64.4	

B	Bsln	90	180	360	540	Days
Mean	43.3	45.0	52.9	52.3	52.6	
SD	9.5	11.6	8.8	5.4	6.1	
Min.	35.2	35.6	37.8	38.6	42.6	
Max.	61.2	64.2	80.0	67.1	62.6	

These activities progressively extended to greater numbers of patients, and promising outcomes were obtained within months. In a survey carried out over 18 months, compared to non-compliant subjects (the control group), patients characterized by an acceptable or a good level of compliance with H-LTOT showed much better control of their condition, with reductions in, for example, chronic

Table 6. Clinical outcomes in subjects included in a 18-month LTOT program (n=34) and in control subjects (n=16)

	LTOT	Controls
M/F	26/8	10/6
Mean age (years ± SD)	67.2±8.4	68.3±5.5
Mean PaO_2 (mmHg ± SD)	53.3±5.7	56.9±7.7
Hospitalizations/year (n)	1.4±0.5 → 0.5±0.2*	1.5±0.8 → 1.4±0.4
Duration, days	26.1 → 9.3*	25.4 → 30.2
Deaths. n	1 (2.9%)	5 (31.2%)

* p<0.01 (Wilcoxon test)

respiratory failure due to severe COPD, and also with significant improvements in their time-courses of PaO_2 (Table 4A, 4B) and $PaCO_2$ (Table 5A, 5B). Moreover, these patients also showed much better clinical outcomes in terms of number of hospitalizations per year and in the duration of hospital stays compared to the control group (Table 6).

Protocols for assessing direct and indirect costs of telemetric LTOT started in those periods and were particularly oriented to comparisons of both the effects and the outcomes of this new protocol versus those of the previous one. Data obtained was very promising and the direct costs of LTOT were easily covered by the savings due to the greatly reduced number and duration of hospitalizations, the reduced number of sick days taken, reduced social and insurance costs, and reduced drug consumption. In particular, the correct use of oxygen in these patients led to a dramatic drop in daily drug consumption: 42% of subjects were shown to be previously taking drugs inappropriately and without any beneficial effect.

The most relevant outcomes of LTOT will be analyzed and commented on in other chapters of this book, together with patient and GP perspectives and discussion of the most recent operative protocols.

In general terms, although a small number of hospital staff and volunteers may effectively be able to maintain the system under routine conditions, such limited human resources cannot adequately manage the daily needs of a large number of patients, particularly in the face of unexpected complications. Despite the good results achieved in Italy with the routine management of LTOT, a small group of specialists immediately switched their attention to other emerging difficulties, the main problem being the ever increasing number of clinically unstable LTOT patients, who were distributed throughout wide or difficult-to-reach geographical regions. Such challenging circumstances were, and still are, so frequent that no medical staff, no matter how large, will ever be able to properly manage the huge number of severe patients at home, which in our case exceeds 160 severe LTOT patients per year.

An innovative model of intervention was needed, founded on a new strategic and technical vision. Considering the solutions that telemedicine can provide, this led to the pursuit of the telemetric option.

References

1. Niewoehner DE, Kleinerman J, Rice DB (1974) Pathologic changes in the peripheral airways of young cigarette smokers. N Engl J Med 291:755-758
2. Medical Research Council Working Party (Stuart-Harris C, Flenley DC, Bishop M) (1981) Long-term domiciliary oxygen therapy in chronic hypoxic cor pulmonale complicating chronic bronchitis and emphysema. Lancet i:681-686
3. Nocturnal Oxygen Therapy Trial Group (1980) Continuous or nocturnal oxygen therapy in hypoxemic chronic obstructive lung disease: a clinical trial. Ann Intern Med 93:391-398
4. Abraham AS, Cole RB, Bishop JM (1968) Reversal of pulmonary hypertension by prolonged oxygen administration to patients with chronic bronchitis. Circ Res 23:147-157
5. Timms RM, Khaja FU, Williams GW (1985) Hemodynamic response to oxygen therapy in chronic obstructive pulmonary disease. Ann Intern Med 102:29-36
6. Calverley PMA, Leggett RJ, McElderry L, Flenley DC (1982) Cigarette smoking and secondary polycythemia in hypoxic cor pulmonale. Am Rev Respir Dis 125:507-510
7. Heaton RK, Grant I, McSweeny AJ, et al. (1983) Psychologic effects of continuous and nocturnal oxygen therapy in hypoxemic chronic obstructive pulmonary disease. Arch Intern Med 143:1941-1947
8. Ashutosh K, Mead G, Dunsky M (1983) Early effects of oxygen administration and prognosis in chronic obstructive pulmonary disease and cor pulmonale. Am Rev Respir Dis 127:399-404
9. Sullivan CE, Berthon-Jones M, Issa FG, Eves L (1981) Reversal of obstructive sleep apnea by continuous positive airway pressure applied through the nares. Lancet i:862-865
10. Howard P (1991) Home respiratory care. Eur Respir Rev 1:563-568
11. Levi-Valensi P, Duwoos H, Giroulle H, Massy-Quelin M, Vonachen P (1974) Etude critique des resultants du traitement ambulatoire par assistance ventilatoire intermittente à domicile et en soins externs à l'hopital de 65 insuffisants respiratoires chroniques graves (38 à domicile, 27 en soins externs). In: Colloque d'Amiens: Traitement ambulatoire des insuffisants respiratoires chroniques graves. Assistance ventilatoire et oxygénothérapie. Boehringer, Ingelheim, pp 467-505
12. Muir JF, Laumonier F (1990) Living conditions of serious chronic respiratory insufficiency patients treated at home on oxygen therapy or assisted ventilation. Lung 168(Suppl):489-494
13. Strom K, Boe J (1988) A national register for long-term oxygen therapy in chronic hypoxia: preliminary results. Eur Respir J 1:952-958
14. Miyamoto K, Aida A, Nishimura M, Aiba M, Kira S, Kawakami Y (1995) Gender effect on prognosis of patients receiving long-term home oxygen therapy. Am J Respir Crit Care Med 152:972-976
15. Weitzenblum E, Chaouat A, Kessler R (2002) Long-term oxygen therapy for chronic respiratory failure. Rationale, indications, modalities. Rev Pneumol Clin 58:195-212
16. Strom K (2001) Oxygen therapy undisputed in severe, but doubtful in moderate, hypoxemia. Comment to meta-analysis of home oxygen therapy in chronic obstructive lung disease. Lakartidningen 98:295-298
17. Wijkstra PJ, Guyatt GH, Ambrosino N, Celli BR, Guell R, Muir JF, Prefaut C, Mendes ES, Ferreira I, Austin P, Weaver B, Goldstein RS (2001) International approaches to the prescription of long-term oxygen therapy. Eur Respir J 18:909-913
18. Hungin AP, Chinn DJ, Convery B, Dean C, Cornford CS, Russell P (2003) The prescribing and follow-up of domiciliary oxygen - whose responsibility? A survey of prescribing from primary care. Br J Gen Pract 53:714-715
19. Morrison D, Skawski K, MacNee W (1995) Review of the prescription of domiciliary long-term oxygen therapy in Scotland. Thorax 50:1103-1105

From National to Regional Criteria for H-LTOT

F. Facchini, F. Trevisan

Oxygen as Medication

Oxygen is not only essential for our respiration, but the Nocturnal Oxygen Therapy Trial (NOTT) and the Medical Research Council (MRC) trial [1, 2] have now documented its use as a medication for patients who are unable to efficiently exchange oxygen from the air to blood circulation. Its prescription is considered when, for different reasons, a person presents with a low alveolar oxygen tension, i.e. a low haemoglobin saturation and arterial blood oxygen partial pressure. The goal of oxygen therapy is in fact to maintain the PaO_2 at >8.0 kPa (60 mmHg) or the arterial oxygen saturation (SaO_2) at 90% [3]. This level of oxygen has been found to be a strong survival predictor [4] and it is thought to be enough to deliver adequate oxygen to the periphery to preserve vital organ function.

Oxygen at room air temperature is a gas and it is delivered as a flow (measured as l/min), added to inhaled air, either via nasal/oro-pharyngeal cannulae or via masks or ventilators. Room air has an oxygen concentration of 21% at sea level. Adding 1 l/min oxygen flow with a nasal cannula is roughly considered to be equal to breathing air with 24% oxygen, 2 l/min to breathing air with 28%, and so on, adding 4% for each additional litre [5].

As a medication, oxygen has side-effects. At very high concentrations it is toxic to lung tissues [6] and hypoventilation [7] is also a risk as oxygen supplementation can increase the ventilation/perfusion mismatch.

Who Can Deliver Oxygen in Italy: Oxygen as Medication and H-LTOT as Service

Article 122 of the Royal Decree 27 July 1934 no. 1265 (of the Health laws) limits drug dispensing to pharmacies. Oxygen is effectively a drug; drug being defined as any substance prepared for therapeutic administration to treat any disease. This means that oxygen can only be delivered through pharmacies, and not through Health Trusts. On the other hand, when oxygen is prescribed for long-term use in chronic diseases, specialist needs and frequent clinical controls have to be taken into account, and this service would be better organised directly by Health Trusts, which necessarily would include drug prescription. The law instituted by the National Health Service (NHS) in Italy (DL 833/1978) specifically indicates that specialist treatments can be given at home, but that specialist home treatments have to be included into day-hospital, domiciliary hospitalisation or domiciliary health care services, referring to hospitals or specialist structures.

Temporary Oxygen Delivery

Usually, short term high "dose" oxygen therapy is considered for acute conditions such as pneumonia, lung embolism, acute alveolitis, asthma attack or exacerbated chronic obstructive pulmonary disease (COPD) and oxygen supplementation has been included in many guidelines as an acute treatment. In most situations, low arterial oxygen partial pressure is associated with normal or low arterial CO_2 partial pressure and risk of hypoventilation is low. However, attention should be given to patients with COPD or when a condition deteriorates, for example where global respiratory insufficiency with CO_2 retention represents a risk of blood acidosis.

Home Long-Term Oxygen Treatment

When oxygen therapy is delivered long-term to COPD patients with respiratory insufficiency (i.e. arterial blood oxygen pressure less than 8 kPa), it improves quality of life and prolongs life expectancy, improves sleep, cognitive functions and emotional status and prevents the progression of hypoxic pulmonary hypertension, especially when used for more than 15 hours a day [1-3, 8-10]. Moreover, H-LTOT has been found to be an effective cost saving strategy as it reduces the number of hospital admissions and exacerbations, offering at the same time a better quality of life to patients [11]. Oxygen prescription has been included in the COPD guidelines of the American Thoracic Society (ATS) and European Respiratory Society (ERS), as well as in the Global Initiative for Chronic Obstructive Lung Disease (GOLD) guidelines [3, 12-18]. The benefits of H-LTOT to all hypoxaemic respiratory patients have been extrapolated from the evidence of its life-saving effects in COPD, and many countries have extended programs for domiciliary oxygen to include patients with other chronic respiratory conditions.

LTOT with Continuous Use

The Italian Drug Formulary (*Guida all'Uso dei Farmaci 2*)[19] has based its recommendations on the Royal College of Physicians Guidelines for home-based oxygen prescription [20] without taking into consideration what has been elaborated internationally [3, 12-16] and nationally [17, 18, 21].

This formulary, which has been sent to all Italian physicians, allows the consideration of LTOT prescription if the following conditions are present:
- COPD with PaO_2 less than 7.3 kPa (55 mmHg) with clinical stability or with PaO_2 between 7.3 and 8 kPa (55-60 mmHg) with concomitant secondary polycythaemia, nocturnal hypoxaemia, peripheral oedema or pulmonary hypertension;
- Pulmonary interstitial diseases with PaO_2 less than 8 kPa (60 mmHg) or if PaO_2 is more than 8 kPa (60 mmHg), along with severe dyspnoea;
- Cystic fibrosis with PaO_2 less than 7.3 kPa (55 mmHg) or with PaO_2 of 7.3-8 kPa (55-60 mmHg) with concomitant secondary polycythaemia, nocturnal hypoxaemia, peripheral oedema;
- Pulmonary hypertension without lung parenchyma involvement with PaO_2 less than 8 kPa (60 mmHg);

- Neuromuscular diseases or skeletal diseases, after specialist evaluation;
- Obstructive sleep apnoea, resistant to continuous positive air pressure ventilation (CPAP) after specialist evaluation;
- Malignant lung tumours or other end stage diseases with severe dyspnoea;
- Cardiac failure with PaO_2 less than 7.3 kPa (55 mmHg) or nocturnal hypoxaemia;
- Paediatric respiratory diseases, after specialist evaluation.

Many differences can be found between these and other national guidelines. When considering COPD patients with arterial oxygen between 7.3 and 8 kPa (55-60 mmHg), the GOLD and *Associazione Italiana Pneumologi Ospedalieri* (AIPO) guidelines are more restrictive as they do not include nocturnal respiratory insufficiency as adjunctive criteria for H-LTOT. On the other hand, AIPO Guidelines tend to widen O_2 prescription in these borderline patients when they present concomitant cardiac ischaemic diseases, right heart failure, and mental deterioration, as this is suggested to benefit tissue oxygenation [12, 17].

If indications for oxygen therapy are met, the patient must be shown also to have stable respiratory insufficiency before H-LTOT can be prescribed: in fact, an acute condition, such as acute pneumonia, can cause respiratory insufficiency that might last longer than the condition itself, in which case H-LTOT prescription is not justified.

The Italian Drug Formulary suggests that the persistence of respiratory insufficiency be evaluated before prescribing H-LTOT, by testing arterial blood gas at least 4 weeks after any acute condition and repeating it after 3 weeks of stability with a thorough evaluation of the respiratory insufficiency (temporary or long-term, risk of hypoventilation) and advice to initiate the treatment in a hospital setting.

AIPO guidelines suggest testing arterial blood gas every 2 weeks for 3 months and discourage the use of the pulseoxymeter for respiratory insufficiency evaluation, unless analysing nocturnal respiratory insufficiency [22].

LTOT with Intermittent Use

It is common to encounter conditions where respiratory insufficiency is not continuous. The Italian Drug Formulary allows the prescription of H-LTOT for intermittent use when patients present with acute episodes of respiratory insufficiency, i.e. acute asthma attacks. This prescription is questionable as it might represent an inadequate or insufficient treatment and delay appropriate medical attention being sought. Moreover, there is no data to suggest that H-LTOT in patients with intermittent hypoxia has any clinical benefit.

More frequently, in advanced respiratory diseases, patients present exercise respiratory insufficiency as measured by the 6-minute walking test or cardiopulmonary exercise test.

It has been reported that significant oxygen desaturation can be registered during common activities such as walking, eating or ablutions [23]. Mechanisms of exercise hypoxia include an increase in airway resistance (normally airway resistance is decreased during exercise), an insufficient respiratory drive with consequent low ventilation, or an increase of the dead space ventilation.

GOLD guidelines suggest limiting H-LTOT to those patients with exercise-induced respiratory insufficiency who also fulfill the continuous use conditions or those patients presenting with severe drops in oxygen saturation during exercise (but no clear values are given to indicate how deep these "severe" desaturations should be). The AIPO guidelines suggest that in those patients with very low FEV1 and PaO_2, especially if signs such as polyglobulia, right heart failure with peripheral oedema or pulmonary hypertension are present [12, 13], intermittent hypoxia should be ruled out. A retrospective study [24] found that DLCO under the limit of 62% of the predicted value was predictive of exercise desaturation, leading to the suggestion of DLCO measurement in patients with exercise respiratory insufficiency.

Anyway, the primary aim of oxygen therapy when prescribed for intermittent use is to improve patient mobility, psychological profile [25] and reduce disease impairment secondary to the exercise respiratory insufficiency. In addition, even if no evidence-based data are available, secondary conditions of hypoxia such as secondary polycythaemia and pulmonary hypertension may thus be avoided.

No indications are given by any Italian national guidelines on how to evaluate the proper oxygen supplementation in these patients. For those patients already on H-LTOT, the NOTT study proposed to increase oxygen flow by 1 l under exercise, but other Authors [26] showed that most patients require higher flow increases during exercise than those suggested by the NOTT study.

Nocturnal H-LTOT Use

About one third of the patients with COPD who present a resting PaO_2 of 8 kPa (60 mmHg) might have oxygen desaturations at night [27], and about half of these patients who have nocturnal desaturations persistently have an oxygen saturation lower than 90% for more than 30% of their sleep. It has been reported that 48% of the patients who received H-LTOT without flow adjustment during sleep still desaturate during the night [28]. Even the NOTT study suggested increasing oxygen by 1 l/min above the resting prescription during sleep or exercise. Worsening conditions in COPD patients during the night might be due to a deteriorating ventilation/perfusion ratio (V/Q mismatch) as well as hypoventilation and presence of sleep apnoea. GOLD guidelines suggest evaluating nocturnal oxygenation, but do not give any indication if and how nocturnal respiratory insufficiency has to be taken into account when prescribing H-LTOT. Nocturnal LTOT is not assessed in the Italian Drug Formulary. Based on expert opinions, AIPO guidelines suggest prescribing H-LTOT if oxygen saturation is under 90% for more than 30% of the recorded period and oxygen delivery at low flows efficiently corrects nocturnal hypoxia [12, 29]. As in the case of intermittent desaturations, nocturnal desaturations should be checked only in those patients where a "reasonable suspicion" exists; that is, patients with very low FEV1 and PaO_2, especially if secondary signs of chronic hypoxia such as polycythaemia, pulmonary hypertension or peripheral oedema are present. It also suggests evaluating nocturnal oxygen needs individually in those H-LTOT patients who have a $PaCO_2$ higher than 45 mmHg, as these patients frequently have greater oxygen needs at night [28].

Besides these points, H-LTOT for nocturnal use is questionable [30]. In fact, the evidence that oxygen is of value during sleep alone (in the presence of normoxia during wakefulness) is equivocal [29, 31, 32], even if some studies link pulmonary hypertension to the occurrence of nocturnal desaturations [33]. For this reason nocturnal monitoring for H-LTOT is rare in other countries, while a survey found that almost 67% of Italian pulmonologists have reported testing patients during sleep [34].

Palliative Indications

It is well known that in clinical settings respiratory physicians are requested to prescribe long-term oxygen treatment for palliative care. There is no value for H-LTOT in these situations, due to costs, side effects and risks of delay in reporting important symptoms to physicians. Both the Italian GOLD guidelines and the Italian Drug Formulary are not clear on this point. They indicate oxygen for intermittent use for severe dyspnoea without evidence of respiratory insufficiency in patients with COPD (GOLD guidelines) or interstitial lung diseases (Italian Drug Formulary). At the same time, directions against the prescription of oxygen therapy as a placebo medication exist (Italian Drug Formulary)!

How to Measure Oxygen Needs: Flow and Duration

The appropriateness of oxygen flow is usually evaluated using the oxygen enrichment test. The goal is to reach a minimum PaO_2 of 8 kPa - 60 mmHg, as this value is a strong survival predictor [4]. First, arterial blood analysis should be done after 30 minutes rest at room air, followed by repeated arterial gas analyses for increasing flow until an arterial PaO_2 of 8.7-10 kPa (65–75 mmHg) is found, avoiding $PaCO_2$ increments that might lead to dangerous pH modifications. Alternatively, the evaluation of basal conditions is suggested and oxygen flow increased until a 90% haemoglobin saturation is reached, thereafter checking acid-basic balance and appropriateness of the oxygen supplementation by arterial blood gas analysis. None of the Italian guidelines clarifies which choice should be favoured, even if the minimal flow necessary to obtain the minimum desired PaO_2 leads to a $PaCO_2$ increase. The ATS/ERS position paper suggests that reversal of hypoxaemia supersedes concerns about CO_2 retention [3], but this might be true only if clinical expertise and technology are available, i.e. in the appropriate clinical setting. Actually, no data are available, as this is often a clinical choice between oxygen supplementation plus ventilation or suboptimal PaO_2 pressure.

Based on the MRC and NOTT original studies [1, 2], continuous oxygen therapy has been recommended for patients with respiratory insufficiency for at least 14-18 hours per day, but recent findings show that pulmonary artery blood pressure increases after 2-3 hours of discontinuation, so AIPO recommends the use of oxygen supplementation for 24, or at least 18 hours.

From National to Regional Criteria

None of the Italian guidelines makes specific recommendations for different regions, as since 1992-1993 (DL 502/92, DL 517/93) the health administration in

Table 1. Bollettini Ufficiali Regionali (BUR) Internet sites (official regional bulletins)

Region	Internet address
Valle d'Aosta	http://www.regione.vda.it/amministrazione/leggi/bollettino_ufficiale_new/default_i.asp
Piemonte	http://www.regione.piemonte.it/governo/bollettino/abbonati/2003/corrente/
Liguria	http://www.bur.liguriainrete.it/
Lombardia	http://www.infopoint.it/bollettini/bollettini_index.htm
Trentino-Alto Adige	http://www.regione.taa.it/giunta/bu/Sommmari_IeII_it.htm
Veneto	http://www.regione.veneto.it/Bollettino+Ufficiale/
Friuli-Venezia Giulia	http://www.regione.fvg.it/istituzionale/bur/bur.htm
Emilia-Romagna	http://www390.regione.emilia-romagna.it/burh/buridx.htm
Toscana	http://www.rete.toscana.it/sett/burt/indexb.htm
Umbria	http://www.regione.umbria.it/canale.asp?id=1441
Marche	http://www.regione.marche.it/bur/home.html
Abruzzo	http://bura.regione.abruzzo.it/
Lazio	http://burl.ipzs.it/burl/burl1.htm
Molise	http://moldat.molisedati.it/web/SommarioRegioneMolise.nsf?Open
Campania	http://www.sito.regione.campania.it/burc/bollettino.htm
Puglia	http://bur.regione.puglia.it/
Basilicata	http://www.regione.basilicata.it/Bur_Bandi_Leggi/bur/
Calabria	http://www.regione.calabria.it/bur/
Sicilia	http://gurs.pa.cnr.it/gurs/
Sardegna	http://www.regione.sardegna.it/bollettino/
Comuni Italia	http://camera.mac.ancitel.it/lrec/

Italy is regionallly controlled. Thus, different political environments might require the adjustment of international or national guidelines to the local situation in order to better answer practical problems met while prescribing H-LTOT. The regional panorama is hard to investigate as it is fragmented, and electronic sources rarely record what was been done before "the Internet era". Although some regions have detailed legislation (Table 1 and Fig. 1), most leave the H-LTOT organisation to the local Health Trust.

Regional Criteria in Valle d'Aosta

Valle D'Aosta is a region composed of only the county of Aosta. Its legislation has taken respiratory insufficient patients' needs into consideration since 1998 (BUR-VdA no. 12 24/03/1998), when it was directed that prescription of H-LTOT materi-

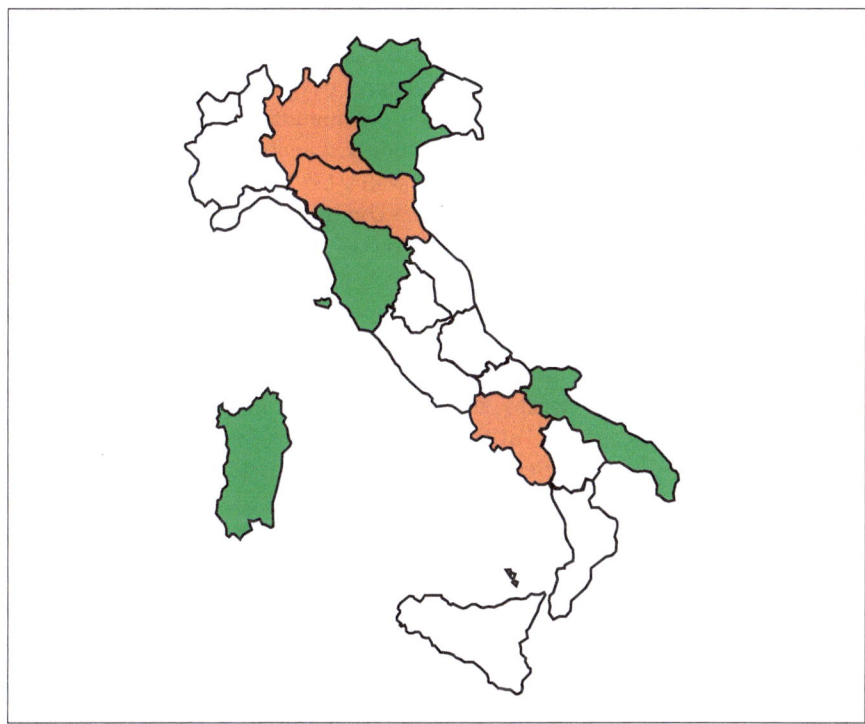

Fig. 1. H-LTOT organisation in Italy: H-LTOT controlled by law or regional Government directives (green), regional guidelines approved or discussed (orange), simple legislation or no data found (white)

als should be done via the local ICU, meaning that H-LTOT is effectively planned by anaesthetists. No guidelines or prescription limits are included in the law. In 2001, oxygen was the second most expensive respiratory medication in Valle d'Aosta and the fifth most expensive of all prescriptions, costing yearly about 437 000 € (the population of the Valle d'Aosta is about 120 000 inhabitants).

Regional Criteria in Lombardia

Lombardia proposed a H-LTOT registry in 1998 [35]. However, no specific regional legislation has been made. Recently, pulmonologists discussed and approved AIPO guidelines without substantial modifications.

Regional Criteria in Trentino-Alto Adige

The autonomous province of Bolzano has clearly defined indications and procedures for long-term oxygen prescription, with a provincial law from 13 March 2000, no. 721. This indicates that the management of patients requiring H-LTOT should be referred to the local Respiratory Service, and the prescribing respiratory specialist should provide a treatment plan in consultation with the general practitioner. The treatment plan provides patient treatment, oxygen flow, timing and means of oxygen therapy, frequency of planned medical and nursing visits, further diagnostic evaluations required and the degree of patient/care giver compliance. H-LTOT can be provided for patients with COPD, interstitial or granulomatous lung diseases, cystic fibrosis, lung resection, primary pulmonary artery hypertension or chronic pulmonary heart disease. When patients with these diseases have respiratory insufficiency, a provisional oxygen therapy is provided and four determinations are carried out within two months, eventually determining the need for long-term therapy. Arterial blood gas analysis findings for H-LTOT prescription should be a PaO_2 less than 7.3 kPa (55 mmHg) or less than 8 kPa (60 mmHg), with the following concomitant conditions: hypoxia during 40 watts exercise or walking test, ischaemic heart diseases (clinical and ECG criteria), cerebral hypoxia, right heart disease (clinical, ECG and pulmonary artery pressure) and polyglobulia with a haematocrit higher than 55%. Nocturnal hypoxia with haemoglobin saturation under 90%, lasting longer than 30% of the recorded sleep is also a criteria for H-LTOT prescription.

When testing oxygen therapy, the goal should be to reach a level over 60 mmHg, with no deleterious $PaCO_2$ increases allowed under this treatment. Minimum prescription for patients with nocturnal hypoxia is 16 hours/day. When patients do not comply with therapy and use oxygen for less than 8 hours/day, oxygen therapy should not be supplied. The mode of oxygen delivery should be customised to each patient by the specialist, taking patient mobility into consideration. If an oxygen concentrator is prescribed, this is provided temporarily by the prescribing centre, then bought through the handicap office, while accessories are provided by the prescribing centre. Electrical costs are refunded to patients by the appropriate Health Trust. Liquid oxygen can be delivered as a service by the local Health Trust or through pharmacies, in which case the Health Trust must refund pharmacies at a price that is 10% lower than the official price fixed for oxygen as medication. This obliges pharmacies to provide assistance within 24 hours for 365 days/year (directly or indirectly). Considering the economic inconvenience for pharmacies, this situation is rarely encountered.

Regional Criteria in Veneto

In late 1986 the region of Veneto was the first in Italy to organise oxygen therapy as a service (circolare no. 44009/6.1.23, 15/12/1986). It directs that patients should access the service through a hospital-based specialist centre: this centre must adopt admission and exclusion criteria, organise initial patient assessment, organise controls, both periodic clinical and home and hospital-based, periodic and emergency equipment controls, in collaboration with the companies who deliver the oxygen to the patient and finally to instruct the patient, care givers and paramedics on how to manage oxygen therapy. At this time, the first regulatory document for H-LTOT management produced by a consensus board of experts was ratified, where all the criteria for accepting or excluding patients were described together with the therapeutic protocols of intervention and follow-up [36].

Regional Criteria in Emilia-Romagna

As far as we know, there is no specific legislation in Emilia-Romagna. In 2000 an organisational model was proposed that was an attempt to solve the problem of lack of data on the number of patients on H-LTOT, inconsistent adoption of clinical indications for prescription of H-LTOT, absence of indications for prescription centres, discrepancies in follow-up protocols, and absence of quality control of private companies delivering oxygen services [37]. Institution of a regional registry for H-LTOT was proposed, defining prescription centres and delivery centres. This registry could be continuously updated, allowing the normalisation of H-LTOT prescription. They suggested the adoption of "international guidelines", i.e. the following clinical recommendations: PaO_2 less than 7.3 kPa (55 mmHg), or less than 8 kPa (60 mmHg) with concomitant right heart failure, pulmonary hypertension, secondary polycythaemia, ischaemic heart disease or clinical signs of brain hypoxia. For H-LTOT, these also included nocturnal desaturation under 90% for longer than 30% of the recorded time and exercise-induced respiratory insufficiency if the patient has improved physical activity with oxygen supplementation. Chronic patients should be confirmed in the following ways: two arterial blood gas morning analyses, with the second test four weeks from the first one. In addition, respiratory insufficiency must be stable and not modified by drug therapies: nocturnal hypoxia has to be evaluated with pulseoxymeter or polysomnography with and without oxygen and exercise and induced respiratory insufficiency should be evaluated with an exercise test (cycloergometer, tread mill, or walking test) with and without oxygen supplementation. It has also been suggested that a follow-up plan should routinely include blood tests, arterial blood gas analysis, electrocardiogram, chest X-ray, spirometry, echocardiogram and medical visits as an outpatient or at the domicile if patients have impaired mobility.

Regional Criteria in Tuscany

Tuscany has had regional legislation on oxygen services since 1988, last revised in 2003 (L.R. 03/03/2003 no. 15). In this regional law LTOT is considered to be any therapeutic plan with oxygen treatment for longer than 3 months in patients affected by chronic diseases with respiratory insufficiency. Oxygen is delivered by the National Health Service with its local trusts via companies who have the duty to report oxygen consumption. Alternatively, oxygen can be delivered through pharmacies (at the same cost). The presentation of a medical statement and clinical documents with diagnosis, exams results, diagnostic procedures and therapeutic prescription are required. Oxygen delivery service is then organised if the documentation follows the diagnostic protocols of the local Respiratory Unit or, in its absence, by other appropriate units. These units have agreed to a protocol that has been included and updated in a document by the Regional Health Council (Respiratory Disease Diagnosis and Treatment Guidelines). H-LTOT is prescribed if patients present a PaO_2 less than 7.3 kPa (55 mmHg) or between 7.3-8 kPa (55-60 mmHg) with concomitant polycythaemia (Ht>55%), ischaemic heart disease, pulmonary hypertension (medium pulmonary artery pressure greater than 3.33 kPa - 25 mmHg) or ECG arrhythmia with heart disease. Before H-LTOT prescription, the clinician should confirm the chronic nature of the respiratory insufficiency by fulfilling the criteria of condition persistence for at least two months and at least three months from the last acute condition, shortening the periods if the respiratory insufficiency is severe (under 6.7 kPa - 50 mmHg). For unstable patients, gas oxygen therapy can be prescribed. Determination of the optimal flow should be done in stable conditions considering also exercise and nocturnal needs, and it is noted that nocturnal evaluation should be done in patients with right heart failure, whereas exercise testing requires not only a pulseoxymeter evaluation but also arterial blood gas analysis performed before and after exercise. When respiratory insufficiency is due only to exercise, then H-LTOT can be prescribed if the patient is active or is included in a rehabilitation program. If nocturnal hypoxia is found, H-LTOT is prescribed when arrhythmia or hypoventilation is documented. Revision of the prescription is suggested yearly and upon any clinical change.

Regional Criteria in the Mid-Adriatic Area

To the best of our knowledge, there are no regional criteria in the mid-Adriatic areas, i.e. Marche, Umbria, and Abruzzo. Each Health Trust has organised its own "oxygen delivery service". This is usually contracted out to a private company. Teramo Health Trust has a private service where oxygen consumption is a required information and some patients are followed with telemetry. Pescara Health Trust has a similar organisation, but with less oxygen consumption controls and without telemetric service. In some Health Trusts, access to the oxygen delivery service is admitted only if the prescribing physician is a respiratory specialist; other Health Trusts, especially those with no easy access to a respiratory centre, require that the internal medicine specialist must be the prescribing physician in order to access the service. There is no rule or strict direction on which type of specialist (pulmonologist or internal medicine) should follow the patient.

Regional Criteria in Campania

No specific legislation about H-LTOT is available in Campania. Pulmonologists have, however, made a proposal to local government where continuous as well as intermittent LTOT is considered.

The continuous H-LTOT indications follow the AIPO guidelines and introduce an additional criteria for neoplastic patients with terminal conditions where a single determination of PaO_2 under 8.7 kPa (65 mmHg) is considered enough for H-LTOT.

For all the conditions, except for terminal neoplastic patients, persistence of respiratory insufficiency must be documented with three arterial blood gas tests made after one hour rest. H-LTOT is prescribed within three to four days if PaO_2 is lower than 6 kPa (45 mmHg), 15 days if PaO_2 is stable, and 30 days if PaO_2 varies more than 10% among the determinations. The optimal flow is identified with an oxygen enrichment test with the goal of a PaO_2 between 8.7-10.7 (65-80 mmHg) without hazardous $PaCO_2$ increases (no $PaCO_2$ limits are given). Controls are planned every three months.

Prescription of nocturnal H-LTOT does not differ from the national AIPO guidelines. When considering exercise respiratory insufficiency, this has to be documented by a pulseoxymeter desaturation under 90% during a walking test (6 or 12 minutes is not specified) or cardiopulmonary exercise test. Oxygen prescription for nocturnal and exercise-induced respiratory insufficiency requires a confirmation test where optimal oxygen flow is determined and efficacy of oxygen administration is proven. Controls are planned yearly.

The regional AIPO document also indicates that H-LTOT should be prescribed only by respiratory specialists within the NHS, limiting the possibility for general practitioners to prescriptions shorter than 30 days.

Regional Criteria in Puglia

Regional criteria have also been clearly defined in Puglia with the aim of giving homogeneous and clear directions when to prescribe, especially in borderline conditions, with patients presenting with hypoxia only in specific situations.

Short-term oxygenation is left to clinical decision and can be prescribed for any clinical situation where it is thought to be necessary. As this is a short-term indication, only the gas form delivered from oxygen bottles is admitted.

LTOT is considered when oxygen supplementation is required and it is delivered for at least 18 hours per day. This therapeutic plan can be prescribed only by respiratory specialists recognised by the national law. In this situation, the regional criteria dictate the prescription of liquid oxygen only for those patients who have the potential for good capacity and performance status, as liquid oxygen allows the patient to move without being wired to a fixed device and consequently improves quality of life. Oxygen concentrators are a more economical option and are prescribed if the patient is unable to have oxygen while outside his/her own domicile. In this situation however, the patient has to cover the electricity expenses.

Regional criteria are then given for LTOT prescription. Puglia has confirmed the AIPO guidelines, specifying that in the case of continuous hypoxia, polycythaemia has to be confirmed by the presence of a haematocrit value of 55%, while chronic pulmonary heart and ischaemic heart diseases should be proved both clinically and electrocardiographically, and pulmonary hypertension should have an echographic evaluation of pulmonary artery medium pressure more than 3.3 kPa (25 mmHg).

When considering nocturnal hypoxia, the Puglia criteria differ from the national guidelines as they introduce comorbidity criteria to the hypoxic limits. For example, LTOT is considered if oxygen desaturation is under 90% for more than 25% of recorded sleep, and there are cardiac arrhythmias caused or worsened by the hypoxia. These criteria are more restrictive than the national guidelines, but still opinion-based. Obviously, as liquid oxygen has been considered for patient mobility, economic reasons dictate concentrator devices as the preferred first choice.

LTOT with intermittent use is suggested for patients with exercise respiratory insufficiency as revealed by an abnormal 7-minute walking test and proved with arterial blood gas analysis at the end of the test. For these patients liquid oxygen is prescribed.

Puglia guidelines also describe how to organise regular controls. These are planned monthly, with arterial blood gas analysis for the first three months, and every three months thereafter. This also facilitates oxygen therapy suspension if clinical conditions improve, upon three months strict observation and arterial blood gas analysis controls.

Puglia guidelines require that the clinician be a respiratory specialist, and must register each patient entering oxygen therapy to allow the better analysis of oxygen consumption and therapy adherence. A form with information for the LTOT registry must be completed for each patient, including patient details, diagnosis, initial prescription, clinical and arterial blood gas analysis control plans.

Regional Criteria in Basilicata

In order to attempt to reduce oxygen costs, the government of Basilicata initially tried to organise H-LTOT as a service (DGR no. 1374/03). No guidelines or prescription criteria were specified in this law, but to access H-LTOT a prescription and therapeutic plan written by a hospital specialist were required.

As the reason for the law was purely economical, pharmacies soon after made a proposal to reduce oxygen cost per litre, in order to avoid income reduction. This proposal was accepted by the regional government (DGR 906 16/04/2004, Razionalizzazione della spesa farmaceutica anno 2004 - Erogazione domiciliare dell'ossigeno liquido ai soggetti aventi diritto - modifiche e revoca DGR 1648/03).

Regional Criteria in Sardegna

A recent survey had difficulties collecting data in Sardegna [38]. In Sardegna, oxygen therapy was regulated initially in 1987 (DGR 45/58, 22/09/1987) and later in 1990 (Direttiva no. 131 06/08/1990) where clinical indications, clinical management and prescription modalities were suggested to attempt to unify very scattered regional H-LTOT prescription praxis. However, regional indications are not fully implemented by the clinicians involved in H-LTOT prescription: the H-LTOT registry planned by this regional directive, for example, was able to collect partial data on oxygen prescriptions only once in 1996.

Conclusions

In Italy, oxygen can be delivered to patients as a medication by any physician through pharmacies, but it requires continuous prescriptions and some types of oxygen are considered inconvenient by pharmacies, as they are not financed by local Health Trusts at the lowest cost. Practical and economical reasons mean that H-LTOT is mostly organised as a service directly by local Health Care Trusts. Italy has had a Regional Health Care System for longer than 10 years. Although some regions have given clear indications to Health Trusts on how to organise the service, most have not. In these cases, the service is organised by the local Trust and guidelines may or may not be given. In this case H-LTOT prescription is left to the physician who may decide differently from the colleague working next door due to lack of data on borderline conditions and different guidelines, mostly based only on "expert" opinions.

Long-term oxygen treatment represents the most expensive therapy for COPD patients and, as nowadays health care might well be limited by available resources, it would be unethical to prescribe an expensive and unnecessary medication. In Italy, about 40 000 patients receive LTOT. The cost per person has been calculated as above 200 € per month [34], but this value varies widely between regions as there are no unique prescription modalities and guidelines differ substantially. It is well known that the cheapest way to deliver oxygen is via oxygen concentrators [34]. Moreover, some recommendations are scientifically questionable and open to interpretation, as in the case of H-LTOT as a "cure" for severe dyspnoea (Italian Drug Formulary and GOLD guidelines).

These conditions have resulted in very variable local situations, from very

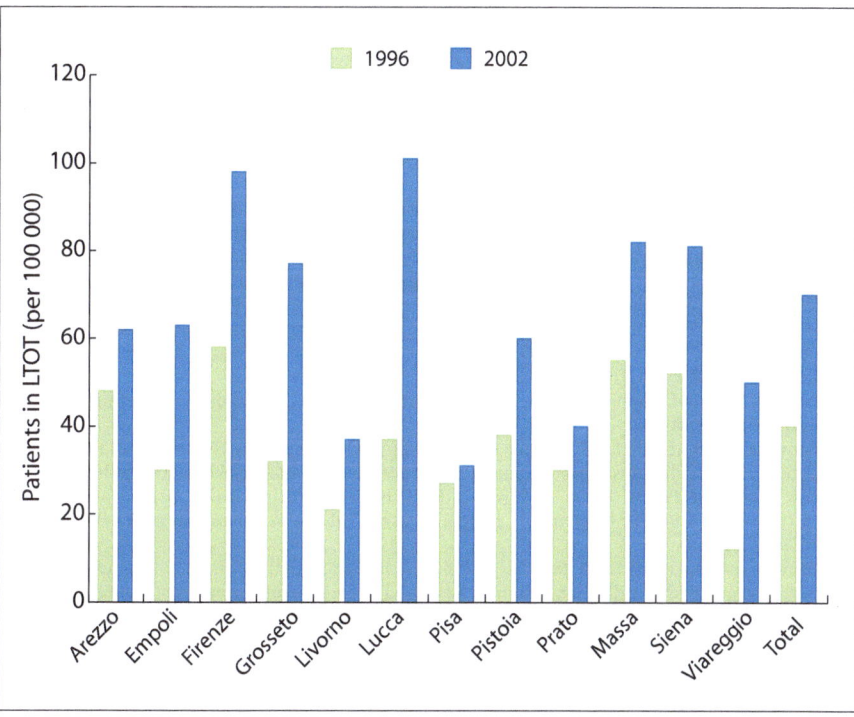

Fig. 2. Number of LTOT patients in Tuscany per 100 000 inhabitants. Data sources: suppliers. Population: ISTAT census data

strict and evidence-based to virtually unlimited prescriptions, with or without periodic controls to evaluate the appropriateness of the prescription itself. Clearly, although it is difficult to evaluate this very fragmented system in detail, even in regions where all official steps have been taken, H-LTOT has very variable outcomes (Fig. 2). In this article, we have suggested some alterations in the system and others might well be drawn from these data. Certainly a lot of work has to be done, both at the national level to unify the guidelines, and at the regional level where health administrations need to establish guidelines for H-LTOT in borderline patients and the best modes of its administration.

References

1. Nocturnal Oxygen Therapy Trial Group (1980) Continuous or nocturnal oxygen therapy in hypoxemic chronic obstructive lung disease: a clinical trial. Ann Intern Med 93:391-398
2. Medical Research Council Working Party (1981) Long-term domiciliary oxygen therapy in chronic hypoxic cor pulmonale complicating chronic bronchitis and emphysema. Lancet 1:681-686
3. Celli BR, MacNee W; ATS/ERS Task Force (2004) Standards for the diagnosis and treatment of patients with COPD: a summary of the ATS/ERS position paper. Eur Respir J 23(6):932-946
4. Skwarski K, MacNee W, Wraith PK, Sliwinski P, Zielinski J (1991) Predictors of survival in patients with chronic obstructive pulmonary disease treated with long-term oxygen therapy. Chest 100(6):1522-1527
5. Shapiro BA, Harrison RA, et al. (1994) Clinical applications of blood gases, 3rd edn. Year Book Medical Publishers, Chicago, pp 169-179
6. Deneke SM, Fanburg BL (1982) Oxygen toxicity of the lung: an update. Br J Anaesth 54(7):737-749

7. Calverley PM (2000) Oxygen-induced hypercapnia revisited. Lancet 356(9241):1538-1539
8. Weitzenblum E, Sautegeau A, Ehrhart M, Mammosser M, Pelletier A (1985) Long-term oxygen therapy can reverse the progression of pulmonary hypertension in patients with chronic obstructive pulmonary disease. Am Rev Respir Dis 131(4):493-498
9. Tarpy SP, Celli BR (1995) Long-term oxygen therapy. N Engl J Med 333(11):710-714
10. Zielinski J, Tobiasz M, Hawrylkiewicz I, Sliwinski P, Palasiewicz G (1998) Effects of long-term oxygen therapy on pulmonary hemodynamics in COPD patients: a 6-year prospective study. Chest 113(1):65-70
11. Dal Negro RW, Pomari C, Micheletto C (1995) Ossigenoterapia domiciliare a lungo termine (OTLT) sotto controllo telematico: aspetti farmacoeconomici. Farmacoeconomia 2(4):43-46
12. American Thoracic Society (1995) Standards for diagnosis and care of patients with chronic obstructive pulmonary disease (COPD). Am J Respir Crit Care Med 152(Suppl 5):S77-S121
13. Siafakas NM, Vermeire P, Pride NB, Paoletti P, Gibson J, Howard P, Yernault JC, Decramer M, Higenbottam T, Postma DS, Rees J (1995) Optimal assessment and management of chronic obstructive pulmonary disease (COPD). The European Respiratory Society Task Force. Eur Respir J 8(8):1398-1420
14. Pauwels RA (2001) Global initiative for chronic obstructive lung diseases (GOLD): time to act. Eur Respir J 18(6):901-902
15. Pauwels RA, Buist AS, Ma P, Jenkins CR, Hurd SS (GOLD Scientific Committee) (2001) Global strategy for the diagnosis, management, and prevention of chronic obstructive pulmonary disease. National Heart, Lung, and Blood Institute and World Health Organization Global Initiative for Chronic Obstructive Lung Disease (GOLD): executive summary. Respir Care 46(8):798-825
16. Pauwels RA, Buist AS, Calverley PM, Jenkins CR, Hurd SS (GOLD Scientific Committee) (2001) Global strategy for the diagnosis, management, and prevention of chronic obstructive pulmonary disease. NHLBI/WHO Global Initiative for Chronic Obstructive Lung Disease (GOLD) Workshop summary. Am J Respir Crit Care Med 163(5):1256-1276
17. Majani U (1995) Direttive AIPO per l'ossigenoterapia a lungo termine (OLT) nei pazienti affetti da insufficienza respiratoria cronica secondaria a broncopneumopatia cronica ostruttiva. Rass Pat App Resp 10:334-344
18. Fabbri LM, Hurd SS (GOLD Scientific Committee) (2003 update) Global Strategy for the Diagnosis, Management and Prevention of COPD. Eur Respir J 22:1-2
19. Ministero della Salute, Direzione Generale della Valutazione dei Medicinali e della Farmacovigilanza (2004) Guida all'uso dei farmaci sulla base del British National Formulary 2. Masson, Milano
20. Report of a Working Party of the Royal College of Physicians (1999) Domiciliary oxygen therapy services. Clinical guidelines and advice for prescribers. RCP Pubblications, London
21. Murgia A, Scano G, Palange P, Corrado A, Gigliotti F, Bellone A, Clini EM, Ambrosino N (a nome del gruppo di studio riabilitazione respiratoria) (2004) Linee guida per la ossigenoterapia a lungo termine (OTLT). Rass Pat App Resp 19:206-211
22. Bellia V, Balzano G, Carone M, De Benedetto F, Del Donno M, Nava S, et al. (1998) Trattamento di base. In: AA.VV. Bronconeumopatie croniche ostruttive: stato dell'arte. Rass Pat App Resp 13:30-39
23. Soguel Schenkel N, Burdet L, de Muralt B, Fitting JW (1996) Oxygen saturation during daily activities in chronic obstructive pulmonary disease. Eur Respir J 9(12):2584-2589
24. Hadeli KO, Siegel EM, Sherrill DL, Beck KC, Enright PL (2002) Predictors of oxygen desaturation during submaximal exercise in 8,000 patients. Chest 122(1): 383
25. Petty TL (1998) Supportive therapy in COPD. Chest 113:256S-262S
26. Guyatt GH, McKim DA, Weaver B, Austin PA, Bryan RE, Walter SD, Nonoyama ML, Ferreira IM, Goldstein RS (2001) Development and testing of formal protocols for oxygen prescribing. Am J Respir Crit Care Med. 163(4):942-946
27. Fletcher EC, Gray BA, Levin DC (1983) Nonapneic mechanisms of arterial oxygen desaturation during rapid-eye-movement sleep. J Appl Physiol 54(3):632-639
28. Plywaczewski R, Sliwinski P, Nowinski A, Kaminski D, Zielinski J (2000) Incidence of nocturnal desaturation while breathing oxygen in COPD patients undergoing long-term oxygen therapy. Chest 117:679-683
29. Fletcher EC, Donner CF, Midgren B, et al. (1992) Survival in COPD patients with a daytime PaO2 greater than 60 mmHg with and without nocturnal oxyhemoglobin desaturation. Chest 101:649-655
30. Zielinski J (1999) Indications for long-term oxygen therapy: a reappraisal. Monaldi Arch Chest Dis 54(2):178-182
31. Fletcher EC, Luckett RA, Goodnight-White S, Miller CC, Qian W, Costarangos-Galarza C (1992) A double-blind trial of nocturnal supplemental oxygen for sleep desaturation in patients with chron-

ic obstructive pulmonary disease and a daytime PaO2 above 60 mmHg. Am Rev Respir Dis 145:1070-1076

32. Chaouat A, Weitzenblum E, Kessler R, Charpentier C, Enrhart M, Schott R, Levi-Valensi P, Zielinski J, Delaunois L, Cornudella R, Moutinho dos Santos J (1999) A randomized trial of nocturnal oxygen therapy in chronic obstructive pulmonary disease patients. Eur Respir J 14(5):1002-1008

33. Fletcher EC, Luckett RA, Miller T, Costarangos C, Kutka N, Fletcher JG (1989) Pulmonary vascular hemodynamics in chronic lung disease patients with and without oxyhemoglobin desaturation during sleep. Chest 95(4):757-764

34. Wijkstra PJ, Guyatt GH, Ambrosino N, Celli BR, Guell R, Muir JF, Prefaut C, Mendes ES, Ferreira I, Austin P, Weaver B, Goldstein RS (2001) International approaches to the prescription of long-term oxygen therapy. Eur Respir J 18(6):909-913

35. Amaducci S, Battaglia E, Rinaldi A, Denti F (1998) Il Registro Regionale dell'ossigenoterapia in Lombardia. Giorn It Mal Tor 52:406-415

36. Dal Negro RW (2000) Long-term oxygen tele-home monitoring, the Italian perspective. Chest 2000 Companion Book, pp 247-249

37. Fiorentini F, Cinti C, Giovannini M, Grandi P, Greco N, Neri M (2000) Proposta di direttiva regionale per la prescrizione di ossigenoterapia nell'insufficienza respiratoria cronica. Rass Pat App Resp 15:58-67

38. Marcias S, Murgia P, Oppo G, Schintu MG, Murgia A, Demurtas R, Coni A, Deiola G, Cordero L, Atzeni R, Camboni S, Greco P (2003) Ossigenoterapia a Lungo Termine e Ventiloterapia Meccanica Domiciliare in Sardegna. Rass Pat App Resp 18:289-296

Systems for Oxygen Delivery

E. Battaglia, S. Amaducci

The current systems for home oxygen delivery consist of:
1. High-pressure cylinders
2. Liquid oxygen systems
3. Oxygen concentrators

At present, the use of high-pressure cylinders is very rare, because this system expires after a short time and it is very costly. For this reason it is used in the hospital or at home in cases where treatment of respiratory failure is of short duration.

High Pressure Cylinders (Gaseous Oxygen)

The first medical oxygen cylinder was manufactured in 1888 in the USA. By the turn of the century, the American Federal Government had established the Interstate Commerce Commission to be in charge of regulating the safe transportation of cylinders, a service transferred to the Department of Transportation (DOT) in 1967 [1].

A high-pressure oxygen cylinder consists of a seamless cylinder of alloy steel, carbon steel or aluminium, a pressure-relief device and a cylinder valve (Fig. 1).

The cylinders have internal volumes (nominal or water volumes) ranging from 1 to 45 litres. The more common sizes are described in Table 1.

The cylinders are fitted with a mechanism that allows the gas to escape if the pressure increases as a result of adverse conditions, such as extreme heat.

Every cylinder uses a direct-acting

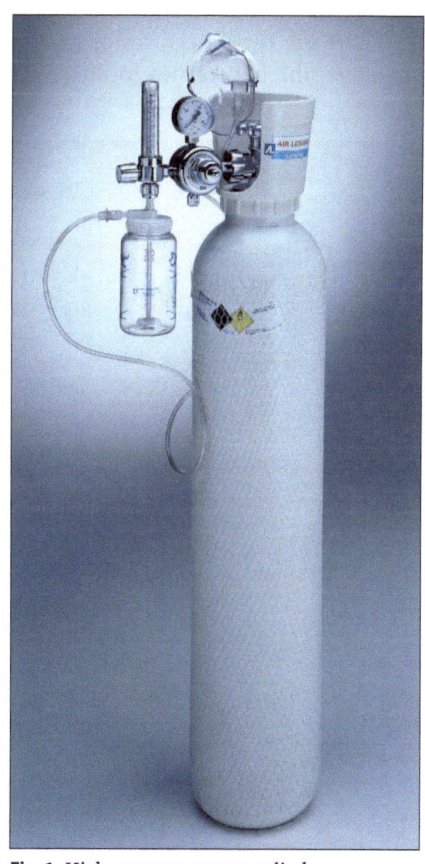

Fig. 1. High-pressure oxygen cylinder

Table 1. Technical characteristics of high-pressure oxygen cylinders

	Capacity				
	500 l	1000 l	1500 l	3000 l	6000 l
Geometric capacity (l)	2	5	7	14	27
Height (mm)	312	480	600	800	1050
Diameter (mm)	110	140	140	204	204
Full weight (kg)	3	8	10	23	35

valve; that is, a type of needle valve, a one-piece mechanism in which the rotation of the handwheel directly seats or unseats the threaded valve. The inlet of the cylinder valve assembly is threaded into the cylinder neck. These inlet threads have been standardised.

The outlet of the cylinder valve assembly is threaded and is the means of attaching the regulator, which reduces the cylinder pressure to working pressure (Fig. 2) [1].

High-pressure cylinders must be white with a white head, according to the law, because they contain therapeutic oxygen [2].

There are two categories of markings that are required to appear on oxygen cylinders: the first relates to the construction of the cylinder itself, whereas the second relates to the oxygen contents. They are generally found stamped on the neck of the cylinder or on a label attached to the cylinder which shows the type of cylinder manufactured, a serial number, the manufacturer's trade mark or identifying symbol and, also, the month and year of the final inspection after manufacture, followed by retest dates [2].

For correct use, valves must be opened very slowly with care, turning the hand-grip anti-clock wise (Fig. 3).

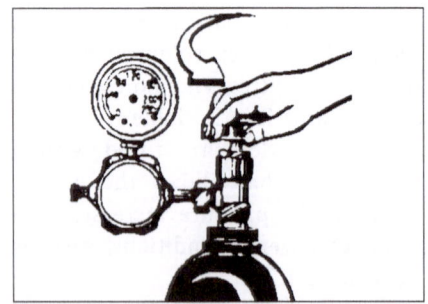

Fig. 2. High-pressure oxygen cylinder security valve   **Fig. 3.** Opening the high-pressure oxygen valve

Table 2. Autonomy of high-pressure cylinders

Prescribed flow	Autonomy (h)	
	3000 l cylinders	1000 l cylinders
1 l/min	45	14
2 l/min	20	7
3 l/min	15	3
4 l/min	10	2
5 l/min	8	1

It is necessary to read the instructions connected to every system carefully.

High-pressure cylinders must not be turned upside down and some models must be chained to fixed surfaces. The cylinder is full when the gauge shows 200 kg/cm^2 (or bar).

Nowadays, cylinders with different capacities are available: 2, 5, 7, 15 and 20 litres, with an autonomy depending on the flow rate of oxygen/minute (Table 2) [2].

When the cylinder is opened, the flow-meter must be adjusted until the prescribed flow is reached (Fig. 4).

Medical oxygen cylinders that are manufactured in accordance with DOT specifications are safe when handled correctly.

The following section lists recommendations for safe home use of oxygen cylinders (Table 3) (Fig. 5) [2]:

- Never allow oil, grease or other readily combustible substances to come into contact with cylinders, valves, regulators, gauges, hoses or fittings. Oil and certain gases such as oxygen or nitrous oxide may cause an explosive compound to form.
- Never lubricate valves, regulators, gauges or fittings with oil or any other combustible substance.
- Cylinders should not be handled with bare hands, gloves or other clothing that contain grease or oil.
- When tank valve protection caps are supplied, they should be secured tightly in place at all times except when the tank is in use.
- Freestanding cylinders should be properly chained or supported in an appropriate cylinder cart or base.
- Cylinders should not be supported by or be in the proximity of radiators, steam pipes, or heat ducts. Cylinder container pressure will rise if heated. Pressure-relief devices are sensitive to pressure. If the relief device breaks, the contents will be discharged into the room and may cause a fire.

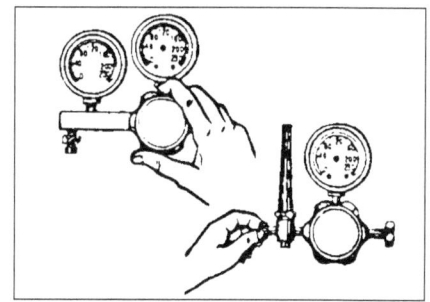

Fig. 4. Adjustment of the flow-meter

Table 3. Recommendations for safe home use of oxygen cylinders

---

• Open the valve very slowly without forcing it

• Use only specified flow-meters and pressure-relief devices

• Do not remove the protection valve caps

• Close the valve very slowly, without force at the end of use

• For any problem call the manufacturer

• Fix the cylinders to surfaces (only for some models)

• Do not smoke

• Remove all easily inflammable substances from the area in which the oxygen is located (oil, lubricants, petrol, hydrocarbons, wood, paint, tar)

• Remove any fire source (flames, sparks, matches, lighters, heat source, bumping)

• Never grease or lubricate the devices that contain the oxygen (taps, valves, connections, piping)

• Only store and use oxygen in ventilated areas

• Keep equipment in an upright position

• Do not remove any components of the unit

• The length of the oxygen cannula is 10 meters at the most: do not try to extend it

• Oxygen flow can be checked by putting the cannula or the mask in a glass of water

• Turn off the cylinder when not in use

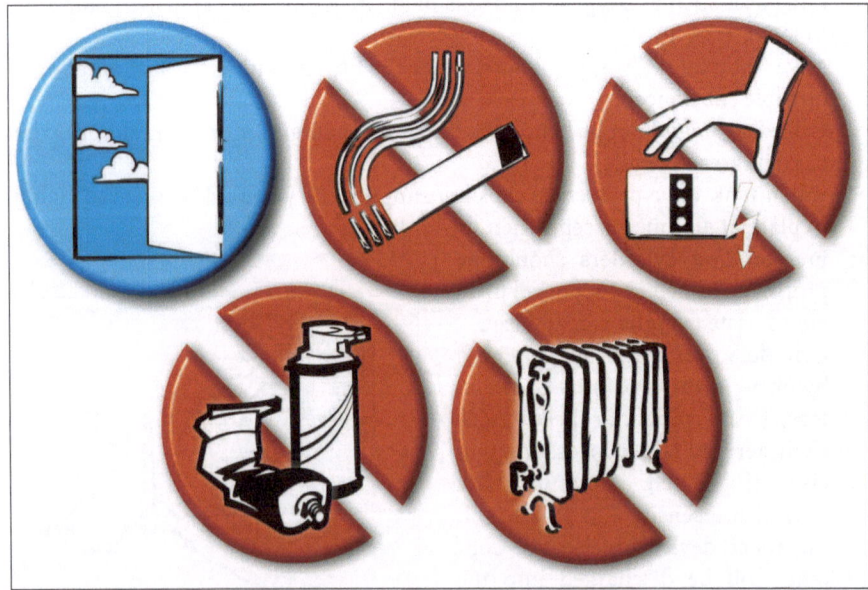

Fig. 5. Recommendations for use

- Never drop cylinders or permit them to bump violently against each other violently.
- Avoid dragging or sliding cylinders.
- Do not remove valve protection caps until ready to empty contents or to connect to a manifold.
- Never allow gas to enter the regulating device suddenly. Always open the cylinder valve slowly.

Liquid Oxygen Systems (Cryogenic Reserve Tanks)

There are several liquid oxygen systems currently on the market; they provide economical and convenient sources of high-volume oxygen. Cryogenic reserve tanks, while varying in design and mechanical systems, are similar in principle.

Oxygen enters the liquid state at or below -183 °C at 1 atmosphere, acquiring a light-blue colour. The usefulness of its liquid state comes from the fact that liquid oxygen occupies 862 times less volume than gaseous oxygen. This allows relatively small volumes of liquid oxygen to provide high flow rates of gaseous oxygen to a patient. In fact, a litre of liquid oxygen stored at 1.5 bar yields 873 litres of gaseous oxygen [1].

Liquid oxygen is stored at home in a reservoir unit known generically as a base or mother unit. It consists of a stainless steel inner vessel that contains the liquid and an outer vessel; the two vessels are separated by a partial vacuum [2]. The inner vessel is generally wrapped in a reflective material to reduce heat transfer by thermal radiation. The vacuum helps to maintain the low temperatures by reducing convection and the separation of the inner and outer vessels reduces heat transfer by conduction. Liquid oxygen transfer occurs in response to a pressure gradient established between the supply vessel and the reservoir unit. The supply vessel is typically pressurised between 50% to 100% higher than the reservoir pressure.

The liquid is introduced to the reservoir unit by means of a supply line that mates with the female quick-connect adapter. The liquid flows through the quick-connect and fill-tube into the inner vessel. This flow will only occur when the vent valve is opened. Initially, a good deal of the liquid entering the unit evaporates and escapes from the unit through the vent valve because the internal components are warm. As the filling continues, these internal components cool and more liquid remains in the unit [1]. There will be additional oxygen loss at this point as a result of liquid displacing the gaseous oxygen. When the inner vessel is full, liquid oxygen spurts out the vent valve. The filling process will end when the vent valve is closed. The pressure and temperature of the oxygen are linked, but this relationship is only valid for a liquid that is balanced or saturated. Balance is only reached when the entire liquid phase has reached the temperature of the gaseous phase.

When the fluid warms up, a rise in pressure occurs naturally with the evaporation of a small volume of liquid oxygen. A valve limits the pressure to 1.5 bar. A rise in temperature slowly develops with the natural entry of heat. A drop in temperature occurs with the progressive evaporation of liquid oxygen. This evaporation consumes thermal energy. It is important to understand this phenomenon because

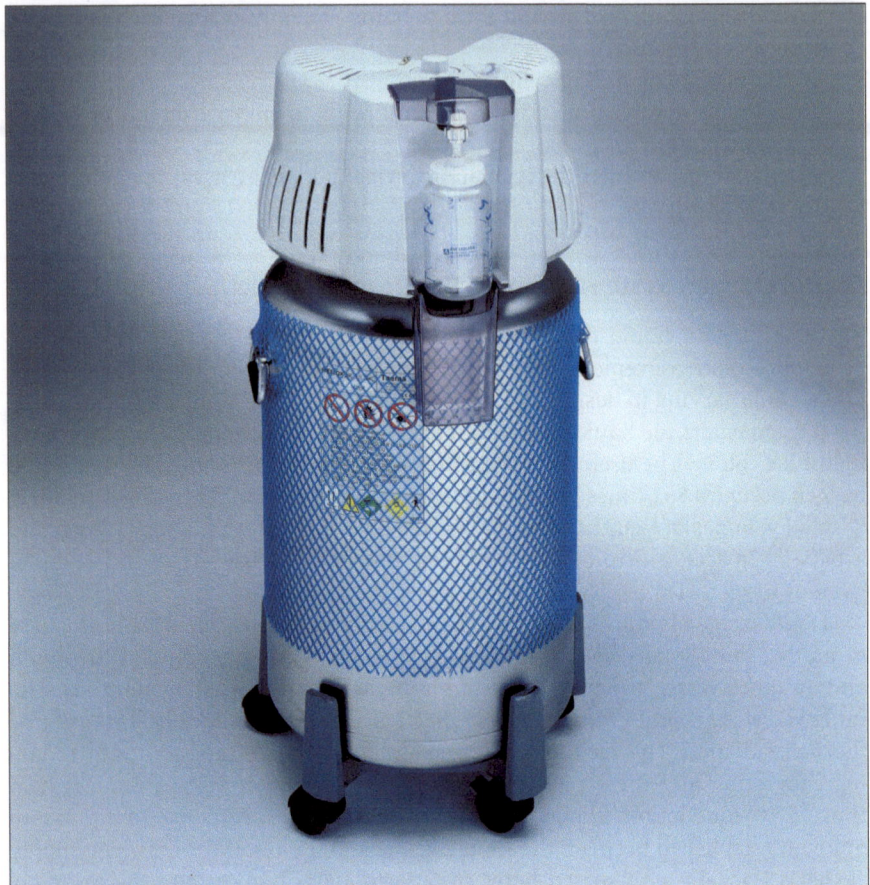

Fig. 6. Reserve tank

the refilling of a reserve tank with a fluid that is too cold triggers a rapid pressure drop when the apparatus is used. This phenomenon disrupts the flow rate and this disruption can last up to several hours following the liquid oxygen delivery. On the contrary, refilling of the tank with a fluid that is too hot triggers significant losses due to the evaporation that occurs during the gradual cooling of the fluid.

The liquid oxygen container was modified to allow both acquisition and storage of data in terms of calculation of both oxygen consumption, reserve and the trend of compliance of the patient to oxygen therapy [3].

The system is composed of two units [2]:

- **the reserve tank (base unit or mother unit)**, the movement of which is facilitated by castors attached to the base; it has a capacity of 20, 32 or 44 l and a full weight no more than 70 kg (UE rules) (Figs. 6, 7)

- **the portable tank** (*stroller*) with a capacity of 0.5 or 1.2 l and a weight of about 3 kg when full; maximum flow of 6 l/min or 15 l/min; it provides great mobility with considerable oxygen autonomy (e.g., 7 hours of autonomy at a flow of 2 l/min with the 1.2 l portable tank) (Table 4) (Figs. 8, 9) [2].

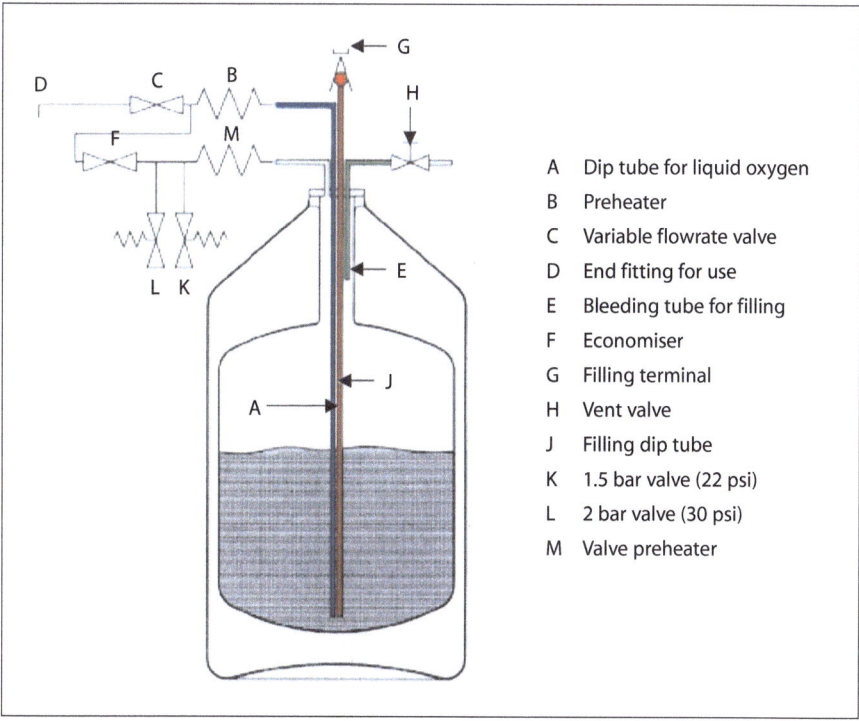

Fig. 7. Structure of a stationary liquid oxygen container

A   Dip tube for liquid oxygen
B   Preheater
C   Variable flowrate valve
D   End fitting for use
E   Bleeding tube for filling
F   Economiser
G   Filling terminal
H   Vent valve
J   Filling dip tube
K   1.5 bar valve (22 psi)
L   2 bar valve (30 psi)
M   Valve preheater

The level of liquid oxygen stored in the reserve tank can be displayed, on request, by an electronic LED or by an LCD indicator (Fig. 10), powered by an alkaline battery located within the indicator itself and electrically connected to a capacity gauge. This gauge has coloured sections (red, yellow and green); the red colour shows that the unit is almost empty, yellow shows that the tank is on reserve and green that the tank is full [2].

Table 4. Cryogenic tank technical characteristics

	Companion LL (Tyco)	Companion C41 (Tyco)	Freelox 44 (Taema)	Penox 40 (Penox)	Liberator 30 (Caire)	Stroller 1.2 L (Caire)
Liquid volume (l)	31	41	40	40	31.20	1.2
Gaseous volume (l)	25 600	33 756	32 600	33 600	27 200	1026
Height (cm)	101.6	95.9	95	81.3	75.0	34.3
Diameter (cm)	36.1	36.2	36	40.6	35.6	Elliptical
Empty weight (kg)	26	27.2	24	24.4	20.4	2.3
Full weight (kg)	61.2	71.6	70	70	54.4	3.6
Autonomy at 2 l/min (h)	-	281	270	280	199	8

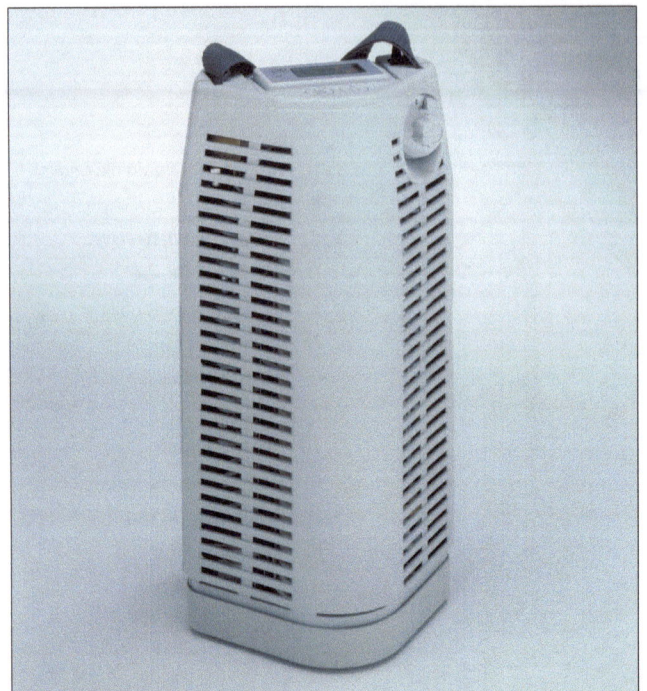

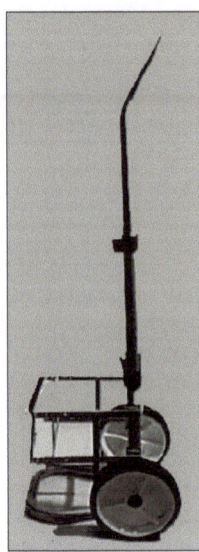

Fig. 9. Stroller cart

Fig. 8. Portable tank (stroller)

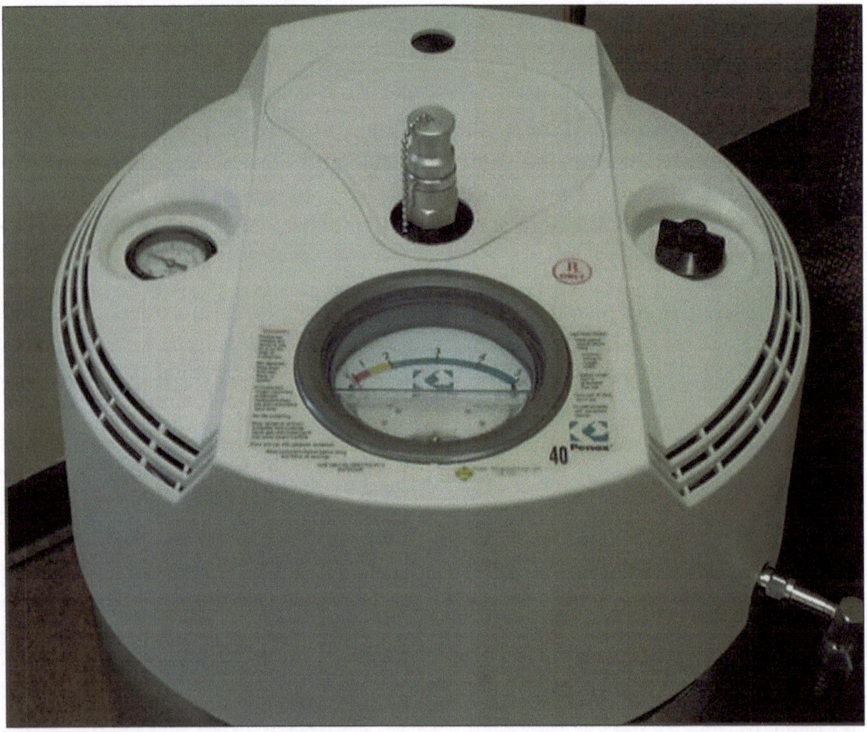

Fig. 10. Level indicator of the reserve tank

This system allows patients and caregivers to monitor the situation over time. Therefore it is necessary to verify the level of liquid oxygen daily and, if it is less than a quarter of the total capacity, to request a refill.

The reserve tank is supplied with the following [2]:

- A female quick-connect for the filling of portable unit
- A button for disengaging the portable unit
- A flow selector
- A humidifier (Fig. 11)
- A condensation collector
- A base with casters.

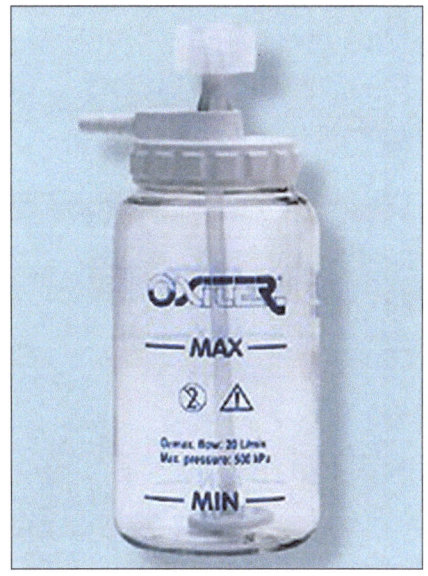

Fig. 11. Humidifier

To start the reserve tank it is necessary to put the condensation collector on the support, connect the humidifier to the oxygen exit link, fill the humidifier with distilled water until the marked level by unscrewing the glass, connect the interface with the humidifier and select the prescribed oxygen flow.

It is periodically necessary to throw out the condensated water from the collector. Minor leaks of oxygen are tolerated and are revealed as rustling or whistling sounds.

The **portable unit** allows the patient greater mobility and it is refilled by plugging it into the reservoir unit.

All portable units are supplied with the following [2]:

- An indicator of level (LED electronic or with an integrated balance, started simply by lifting the portable unit by the belt nearest the indicator)
- An interface connector
- A flow selector
- A battery box
- A unit vent
- A condensation collector.

To fill the portable unit it is necessary to plug it into the female quick-connect on the reservoir tank. The connector may be mounted either on the top or side of the reservoir unit (Figs. 12, 13). The mating connector on the portable unit can be filled in one of two positions. When connected to the top, the portable unit is inverted, filling top to top. Side-mounted connectors fill the portable unit in an upright position.

The patient or caregiver should be taught the following basic steps in order to fill the portable unit:

- Make sure that there is enough liquid oxygen in the reservoir to fill the portable unit;

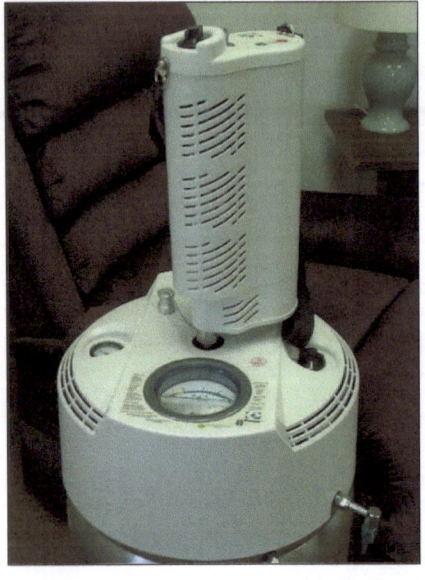

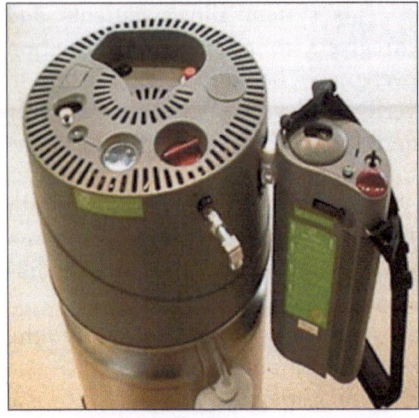

Fig. 13. Refilling the portable unit (connector on the side of the unit: especially for patients with restricted movement)

Fig. 12. Refilling the portable unit (connector on the top of the unit)

- Check the connectors on both units to make sure that they are clean and dry. Moisture on these connectors could cause the connectors to freeze together;
- Connect the portable unit to the reservoir according to the manufacturer's instructions. The flow rate controller should be turned off;
- Open the portable unit vent. Allow the portable unit to fill until the vent valve begins to pass liquid oxygen instead of gas. Close the vent valve;
- Disengage the portable unit according to the manufacturer's instructions.

During the use of the cryogenic tank, some problems may occur as seen in Table 5 [2].

Systems for oxygen delivery and interfaces must periodically undergo maintenance by the manufacturer and by the patient or caregiver.

Table 5. Problems that may occur during use of the cryogenic tank

Observations	Causes	Solutions
Flow rate too low	Internal pressure too low	Check for insufficient pressure
	Intake filters of flow valve	Change the valve intake filters
	obstructed	Perform the flow valve cleaning
	Hole in flow valve obstructed	procedure
	Frozen liquid on plug	Change the flow valve
		Drain the reserve tank and pipes
No display (for LED indicator)	No electricity supply	Call manufacturer
	Indicator not working	
Nasal cannula or connecting catheter are full of water	A lot of condensation is produced	Empty the humidifier and open the flow of reserve tank until the pipe is dry

Checking procedures should be carried out daily, weekly and monthly [2].

Daily maintenance
- Remove the humidifier
- Rinse it with water
- Put distilled water into the humidifier until the level indicated
- Connect the humidifier with the reserve tank
- Wipe the connections of the reserve tank to the portable unit with a clean and dry cloth.

Weekly maintenance
- Remove the humidifier
- Throw away water
- Rinse it with water and a liquid detergent (a slightly foaming liquid soap) to avoid calcium deposits
- Rinse with water
- Dry and connect to reserve tank.

Monthly maintenance
- Disinfect equipment (humidifier, condensation collector), immersing them for 10 minutes in a detergent (DO NOT USE INFLAMMABLE SUBSTANCES LIKE ALCOHOL)
- Rinse equipment well.

Finally, it is very important to give the patient and caregiver some general safety instructions. First of all, to avoid burns, the cold or frosted areas should never be touched. In order to prevent any fluid leaks, the tanks must be kept in an upright position. Electronic devices, such as mobile phones, CB radios, microwave ovens etc., should be avoided in the vicinity of the cryogenic tank. Oxygen is not an inflammable gas but does accelerate the rate of combustion of other materials. In order to prevent any risk of fire, the system should be positioned at least 1.5 m away from any smokers, flames, electrical appliances or inflammable products, such as oils, lubricants, solvents, aerosol canisters etc. Liquid oxygen is extremely cold (-183 °C), so the parts of the tank that come into contact with liquid oxygen, when the tank or portable unit are being filled, may cause burns if they come in contact with the skin.

It is also important not to leave the portable tank connected to the reserve tank; lock the flow rate selection buttons whenever the machine is not in use; position the system in a ventilated area; keep the tanks in an upright position at all costs.

Liquid oxygen can easily be adsorbed by porous substances, such as cloth, wood or rubber foam and therefore may cause sudden combustion.

Fuel mixed with liquid oxygen can explode when slightly bumped or for other causes, such as friction or sparks.

Hydrocarbonated oils and lubricants are particularly dangerous when oxygen is present since they can spontaneously flare up and burn with frightening speed. They must never be used as a lubricant for equipment that works with oxygen or over-oxygenated air. However, special lubricants that are compatible with oxygen can be used under certain conditions.

It is important to avoid the following incorrect usages of oxygen (Table 6) [2]:
- Supply for pneumatic tools
- Ventilation for people
- Air cooling or renewal in confined spaces
- Dust removal from benches, machines and clothes.

Liquid oxygen is the best system for oxygen delivery for patients who still have a good level of autonomy or mobility outside the home; it is also the best system in case of oxygen desaturation during effort [4].

Table 6. General safety instructions for cryogenic reserve tanks

---

• Do not smoke

• Do not leave the portable unit connected to the reserve tank during therapy

• Lock the flow-rate selection buttons whenever the machine is not in use

• Fill portable unit in a ventilated area and on a non-flammable surface (cement, brick paving or concrete)

• Do not leave the cryogenic tank during filling of portable unit

• If you cannot close the vent valve of portable unit, do not force; it may be due to frost→take away the stroller by pressing on the button to disengage portable unit. The oxygen flow will stop immediately. Turn off the vent valve when the frost disappears

• Avoid any impact or exertion of abnormal pressure on frozen parts

• Restrict ice formation by drying removable parts to prevent them from getting blocked

• Avoid sudden leakage of fluid at the end of the filling procedure

• Liquid oxygen may cause burns when it comes in contact with the skin

• Store and use oxygen tanks in ventilated areas

• Do not keep portable unit under clothes or rolled up in a rag

• Do not roll or tilt the tank when moving it

• If the stroller is used in the car, provide enough ventilation (leave windows open) and avoid rolling of the portable unit (attach it to headrest)

• Liquid oxygen must always be transported in accordance with requirements imposed by national and international regulations currently in force (Fig. 14)

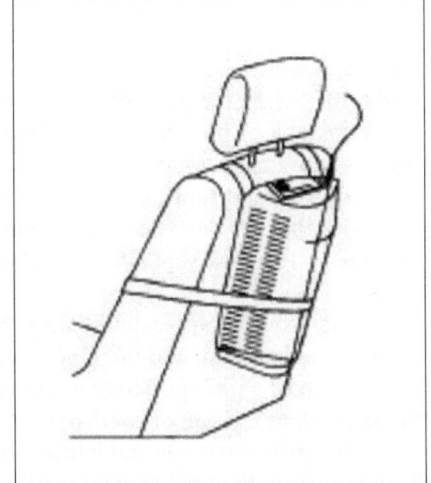

Fig. 14. Attaching portable unit to headrest

Oxygen Concentrators

Oxygen concentrators are electrical devices that separate oxygen from the other gaseous elements in the atmosphere; they collect this separated oxygen into a tank and then deliver the oxygen to the patient via a flow rate control device (Fig. 15) [5].

The concentration decreases with the increase of oxygen flow; in fact, it is possible to reach the best results with a flow of 2 l/min (concentration >95%), while it is not recommended to use it for flow over 5 l/min (concentration <90%) [4, 6].

The most common type of oxygen concentrator uses a molecular sieve material to separate the oxygen from the rest of the air by the process of absorption. The two molecular sieve

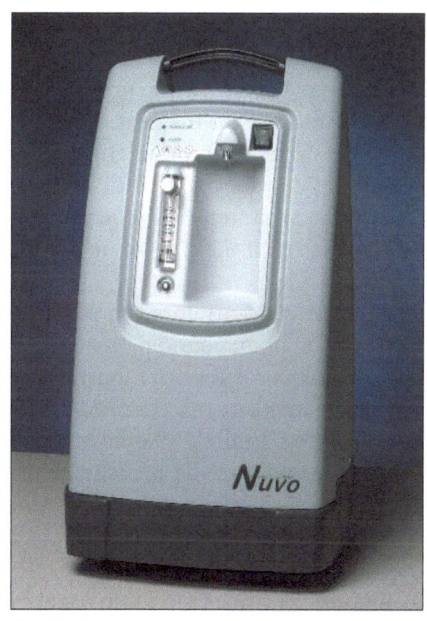

Fig. 15. Oxygen concentrator

beds are the heart of the oxygen concentrator. The term 'pressure swing cycle' refers to the operating phases in which one bed is pressurised to produce oxygen while the other is depressurised to purge the unwanted waste gases.

The molecular sieve material itself is a granular zeolite crystal which has the unique ability to separate gases from each other according to the molecular size and polarity of the gases. In fact, zeolite crystals contain a precisely arrayed network of small, uniform holes. These holes are about 5 angstrom in diameter and together they form the molecular sieve. The particular zeolite in an oxygen concentrator has a preferential affinity for nitrogen, water, carbon dioxide, carbon monoxide and all hydrocarbons, whereas oxygen and minute quantities of argon pass through [5]. In addition to molecular size and polarity, the amount of any particular gas adsorbed is proportional to the partial pressure of that gas, which is why the molecular sieve beds are pressurised.

There is an electronic logic device, such as a printed circuit board or microprocessor that governs the timing of the pressure-swing cycle. As a result of this electronically controlled valving, each sieve bed has two distinct operating phases, the pressurising interval and the depressurising interval. When the first sieve bed enters the pressurising interval, the solenoid directs the air into that cylinder, and a restrictor downstream of the bed builds the air pressure to increase the absorption of nitrogen as the oxygen passes through. The crossover assembly passes the first small portion of this oxygen flow to the product tank for storage and patient use [1]. The remainder of the oxygen is diverted to the second sieve bed to purge the nitrogen absorbed from the previous cycle. As the first sieve bed becomes saturated with nitrogen, the electronic logic device switches the solenoid to the depressurising interval by opening the exhaust to the first sieve bed, allowing backflow to occur in this bed. This reduces the partial pressure of the nitrogen, promoting desorption. This backflow also draws oxygen from the second bed, which is now pressurising, promoting further desorption. This bed is now regenerated and ready for the next cycle.

These cycles are typically timed from 10 to 30 seconds, depending on the manufacturer.

An alarm system will sound an audible alarm if the power to the unit is interrupted or if the electronic logic device senses low system pressure or overheating.

Oxygen concentrators represent the most economic oxygen delivery system, especially in homebound patients [4]. Function requires electric current; they can be used in the car for brief journeys, using the car's lighter. Their weight is about 30 kg. The majority reach a maximum flow rate of 5 l/min, with a graduating scale from 0.25 to 5 l/min [2]. Some models are supplied with an electronic device that constantly analyses the percentage of oxygen distributed. An acoustic or visual alarm shows when the concentrator is not working.

Maintenance should be carried out every 30-60 days and it is particularly important to change filters.

For use warnings see Table 7 and Fig. 16 [2].

Research to improve oxygen delivery systems is ongoing. The most recent innovation is represented by oxygen concentrators that are also able to fill portable oxygen cylinders. This ability greatly reduces the cost and inconvenience of portable systems [5, 7].

There is at least one group working on an oxygen concentrator system capable of producing liquid oxygen while gaseous oxygen is delivered to the patient [5, 7].

Table 7. Oxygen concentrator use warnings

• Do not use multiple sockets

• Do not use extra long cables (danger of stumbling)

• Do not use solvents to clean surfaces; if necessary use damp rag

• Keep away from heat

• Periodically clean the air filter, washing it with water and dry it without direct heat

• Remove humidifier daily, rinse it with water and fill it again with distilled or boiled water until the indicated level

• Wash humidifier with cold water and a detergent every three days

---

Fig. 16. Recommendations for concentrator use

Nowadays, a lot of groups have also developed systems connecting the home unit to the home care company or to the physician by telemetry.

Acknowledgements. Figures 1, 2, 6-8, 15 are courtesy of Taema, ANTONY Cedex, France; Figures 9 and 13 are courtesy of Chart Bio Medical, Sunbury-on-Thames, UK; Figures 10 and 12 are courtesy of Penox, Pittston, USA.

References

1. Lucas J, Golish JA, et al. (1988) Home respiratory care. Appleton & Lange, Norwalk (USA)
2. Amaducci S, Battaglia E, Iuliano A (2003) Dispositivi per la terapia respiratoria. In: Manuale di ausili e cure del paziente geriatrico a domicilio. UTET, Milano, pp 353-377
3. Dal Negro R, Turco P, Pomari G (1991) Progetto di telemetria per l'Home Care respiratoria. Risultati preliminari. Rass Pat App Resp 6(1):111
4. Murgia A, Scano G, Palange P, et al. (2004) Linee guida per la ossigenoterapia a lungo termine (OTLT). Aggiornamento anno 2004. Rass Pat App Resp 19:206-219
5. Kacmarek RM (2000) Delivery systems for long-term oxygen therapy. Respir Care 45(1):84-92
6. Johns DP, Rochford PD, Streeton JA (1985) Evaluation of six oxygen concentrators. Thorax 10(11):806-810
7. McCoy R (2000) Oxygen-conserving techniques and devices. Respir Care 45:95-103

The Interfaces

S. Amaducci, E. Battaglia

Nowadays a lot of interfaces are available for oxygen therapy; these include nasal cannulae, simple oxygen masks, transtracheal catheters, nasal catheters, oxygen devices for tracheostomy, oxygen economizers, Venturi masks and reservoir masks.

Nasal Cannulae

Nasal cannulae represent one of the most simple, economic and likeable systems among the available interfaces (Fig. 1). Their correct usage requires only a small amount of training.

FiO_2 delivered with this system is not accurate because it depends on respiratory rates, tidal volumes and I/E ratios [1]; in fact the first l/min increases the FiO_2 by 3 scores (from 21 to 24%), while the next l/min increase it by 4 scores each (for example 5 l/min allowing it to reach a FiO_2 of 40%) [2].

These small increases are usually enough to improve the arterial oxygen content to acceptable clinical levels. The FiO_2 is inversely related to inspiratory rates: a more rapid inspiratory rate dilutes the oxygen flowing into the nostrils with more room air as well, thereby reducing the FiO_2. The flow is often imprecise: up to a 20% variation is frequent and acceptable [3].

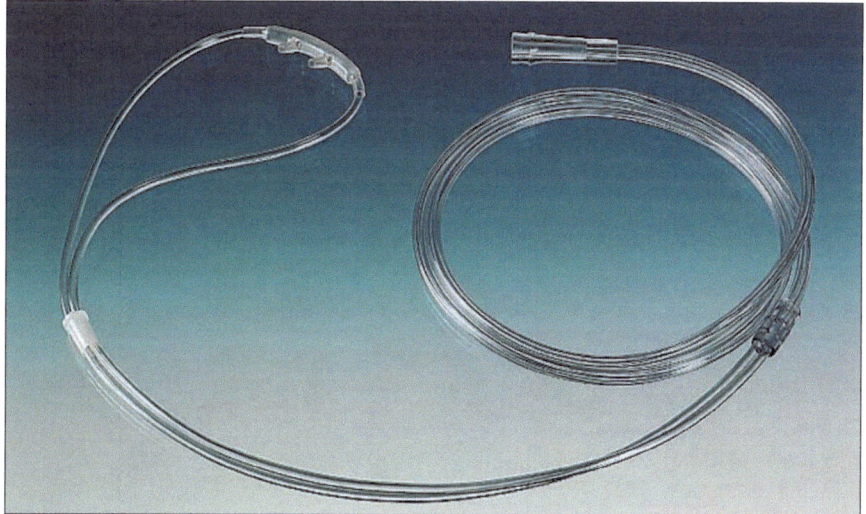

Fig. 1. Nasal cannula

Table 1. Advantages and disadvantages of nasal cannulae

Advantages	Disadvantages

• Low cost
• Little training for use
• Simple to put on the face
• Not uncomfortable
• Allow the subject to talk, to eat, to drink
• Low risk of claustrophobia
• Low risk of inhalation/obstruction
  of airways in case of vomiting
	• Easy dislodgment during sleep
	• Restriction of some daily actions
	  (washing, dressing)
	• Not useful if the patient breathes
	  with open mouth
	• Not useful in case of rhinitis
	  or nasal obstruction
	• Can cause ulcerations of the skin
	  (ears, nostrils)
	• Dryness of nasal mucosa and epistaxis
	• Non aesthetic

Nasal cannulae are also not useful in case of elevated oxygen flow.

In Table 1 advantages and disadvantages of nasal cannulae are shown.

A lot of patients refuse dependence on oxygen for psychological reasons, especially when they are discharged from hospital; for this reason patients tend to try to limit their social relationships and outdoor life.

In order to avoid this, some years ago, oxygen therapy eyeglass frames were put on the market (Fig. 2). They can offer an improvement in quality of life so that the continuous administration of oxygen during the day for several months of the year can become acceptable for these patients.

These oxygen therapy frames are both unobstrusive and cheap. They also can be adapted to any kind of lenses, even sun glasses.

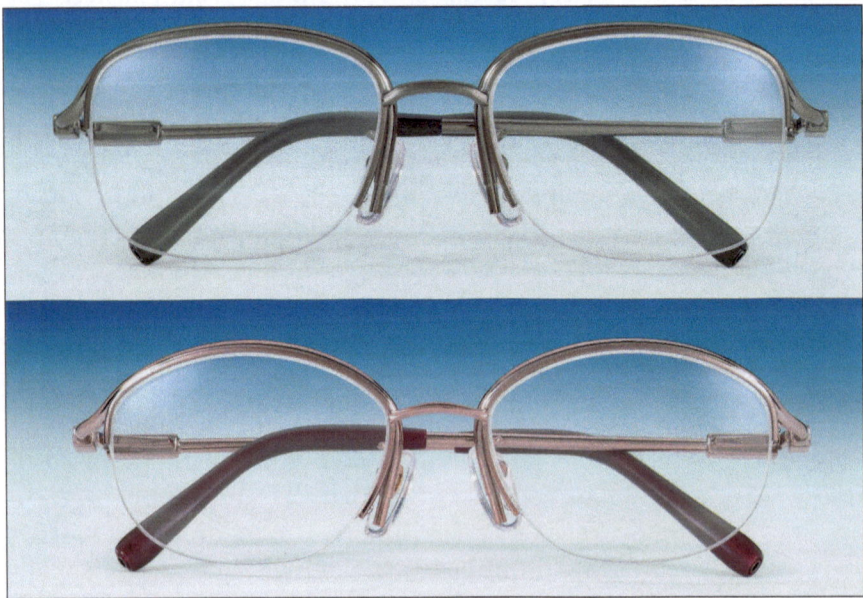

Fig. 2. Oxygen therapy eyeglass frames (Courtesy of Oxy View Inc., Englewood, USA)

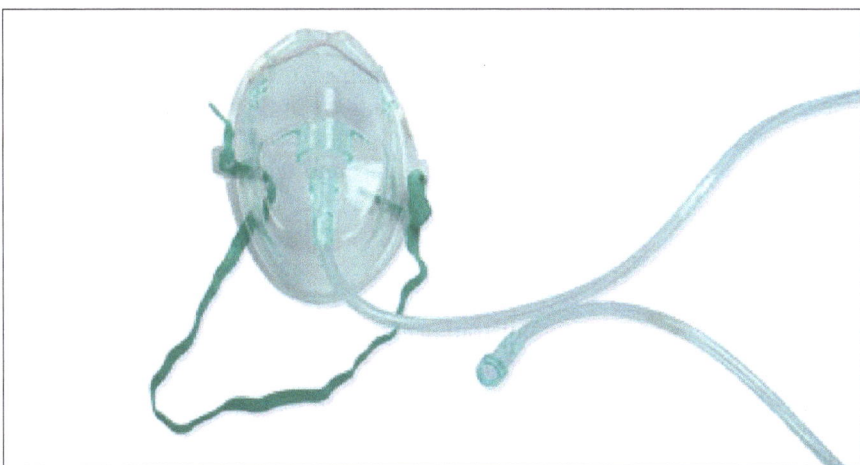

Fig. 3. Facial oxygen mask

Simple Facial Oxygen Masks

These represent a good alternative to nasal cannulae, especially for high delivery oxygen flows. They are used particularly in hospitals; for this reason domiciliary prescriptions are rare. The masks are made of transparent plastic and are provided with a nasal metal clip for greater comfort and better adhesion to the face and are provided with an adjustable rubber band to fix them to the patient's face. They are available in three sizes: pediatric, adult and extra-large (Fig. 3).

The simple facial mask, with a mask volume of 100 to 300 ml, will deliver a FiO_2 of 35 to 55% at 6 to 10 l/min. Supply flows greater than 5 l/min are recommended to eliminate CO_2 [4].

The mask is similar to the nasal cannula in its dependence on ventilatory rates and respiratory patterns in order to reach the desired FiO_2. The mask is useful for patients who are strictly mouth breathers, as well as some patients with extreme nasal irritation or nose bleeding [4]. On the other hand, face masks are obtrusive, uncomfortable and confining, they muffle communication and obstruct eating. They have a lot of disadvantages compared to nasal cannulae; in fact they do not allow eating or talking and they increase the anatomic death space (Table 2). Moreover they are less attractive than nasal cannulae.

Table 2. Advantages and disadvantages of facial oxygen masks

Advantages	Disadvantages
• Less risk of dislodgment • No air leaks from mouth • More accuracy during elevated oxygen flow delivery	• High risk of inhalation in case of vomit • High risk of claustrophobia and aerophagia • High incidence of skin ulcerations • Limited social relationships (talking, eating, drinking)

Reservoir Facial Masks

These are masks supplied by a reservoir in which oxygen flows at 8 to 10 l/min, so that the patient inhales a high concentration of oxygen (Fig. 4). Hence, this system can deliver up to 90% of FiO_2 when the mask is tightly sealed to the face [4]. On the other hand, a tightly sealed mask can be very uncomfortable and thus difficult to tolerate. Higher oxygen concentration also creates a greater risk of CO_2 retention.

Venturi Facial Masks

These masks allow oxygen administration at fixed and established concentrations. Venturi masks, supplied with high oxygen flows, maintain a fixed ratio of oxygen to room air, thus maintaining a constant FiO_2. They allow FiO_2 to be established and are supplied with coloured valves that are interposed between mask and circuit in order to reach an established oxygen concentration.

Typical FiO_2 settings include 24, 28, 31, 35, and 40% [4].

These masks are used more frequently in hospitals; they can also be used at home but in rare cases, for short periods of treatment and under very strict medical control. If not used in the correct way, they cause an increase of carbon dioxide retention.

The different coloured valves allow choice of a different percentage of FiO_2 (Fig. 5) (Table 3).

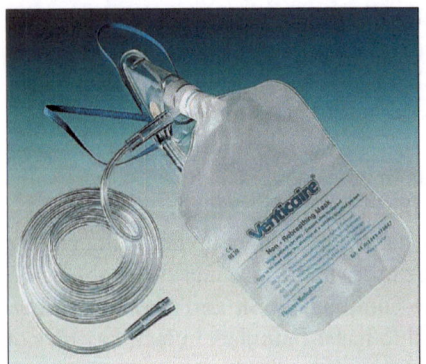

Fig. 4. Reservoir mask

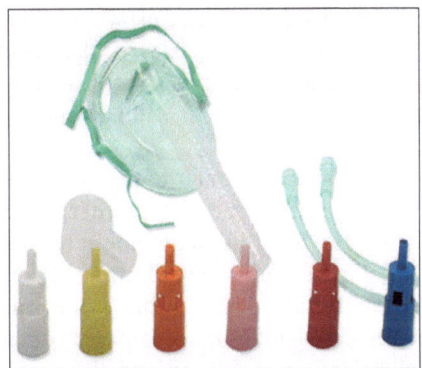

Fig. 5. Venturi mask

Table 3. Venturi facial masks

Colour	FiO_2	Oxygen flow rate
Blue	24%	2 l/min
White	28%	4 l/min
Orange	31%	6 l/min
Yellow	35%	8 l/min
Red	40%	10 l/min
Green	60%	12 l/min

Nasal Catheters

To insert a nasal catheter, plastic tubes are put through the nasal canal to reach the trachea. There are some advantages, if compared to nasal cannulae; these include their stability and the fact that they allow oxygen dispersion and respiratory work to be decreased.

There are also some disadvantages, such as they are very uncomfortable and they often need to be fixed to skin with plasters. It is also necessary to humidify oxygen to avoid the formation of mucous plugs (Fig. 6). For this reason they are avoided for long domiciliary uses.

Transtracheal Oxygen Therapy

Transtracheal oxygen therapy (TTOT) is a method of long-term continuous oxygen delivery, using a catheter inserted into the trachea through a tracheocutaneous tract [5].

Heimlich's original technique consisted of administering oxygen directly into the trachea via a 16-gauge intravenous catheter that was inserted between the second and third tracheal rings and sutured to the skin [6].

TTOT is recommended in cases of refractory hypoxemia, intolerance to nasal cannulae (epistaxis, local irritation or allergy), voluntary or involuntary noncompliance (nocturnal dislodgement, aesthetic reasons), the need to improve mobility by reducing oxygen flow and loss of olfactory sensation [5].

Direct oxygen administration into the trachea resulted in a number of benefits, not the least of which was a 50% to 60% oxygen saving [7]. The most important benefit of transtracheal oxygen therapy is the ability to conceal the oxygen catheter under clothing; portable oxygen used by the patients can be half the size normally required with nasal cannula use and the procedure has allowed many patients to return to work or increase their time outdoors.

Contraindications are represented by herniation of the pleura at the insertion site (emphysematous bleb), coagulapathies, severe comorbid conditions or terminal illnesses, impaired cough reflexes, lack of willingness, lack of ability of patient or family to take care of the catheter, inability to communicate and upper airway obstruction [8].

A variety of TTOT catheters are

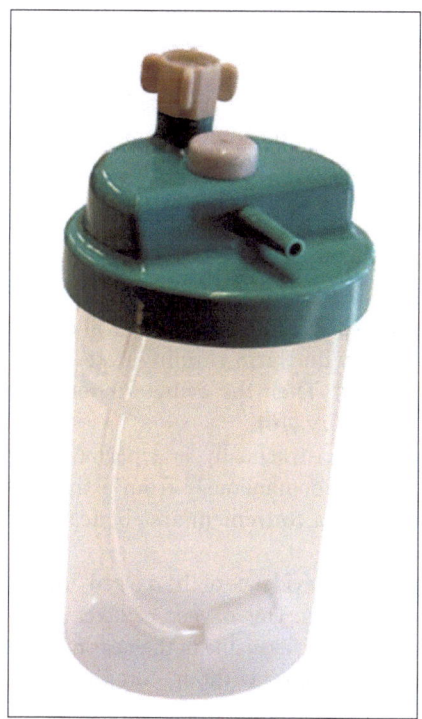

Fig. 6. Oxygen humidifier

available. Clinical studies favour the use of a multi-step procedure kit to promote standardization of the technique, improve patient's adaptation and minimize complications. For high-flow oxygen therapy (>4 l/min), a permanent catheter with multiple fenestrations is preferred. This reduces back-pressure and accidental disconnection of oxygen tubes. The catheter should be more than 3 mm in diameter and long enough so that the distal tip will be 2-3 cm above the carina [5].

Proper patient and family training is mandatory prior to the TTOT procedure.

The multi-step TTOT procedure involves aseptic catheter insertion into the trachea, under local anaesthesia using the Seldinger technique. During the first week after insertion, the initial catheter allows tract formation. No oxygen is delivered during this period. The initial catheter is replaced with a softer, single-port catheter for oxygen delivery. This is left in place for 8 weeks and cleaned without removal. The final step involves replacement of the second catheter with a softer fenestrated catheter which can be replaced and cleaned by the patient through a mature tracheocutaneous fistula [5].

The use of antibiotics, cough suppressants and pain medications is advocated during the first week. The patient's competency must be evaluated at every visit which should be at least every three months for the first year after the TTOT insertion. The TTOT catheter should be replaced according to the manufacturer's recommendations.

TTOT produces therapeutic levels of blood oxygen content with lower flow rates than those needed in other oxygen delivery systems, at rest as well as during exercise [9]. Minute ventilation and the work of breathing are reduced. Exhaled minute ventilation and the carbon dioxide pressure in arterial blood remain unchanged. The metabolic work performed by the inspiratory muscles and the diaphragm is also reduced. Exercise endurance, assessed by the 6-minute walking test, is better with TTOT than with oxygen via nasal cannulae [9]. TTOT may confer a greater survival benefit than does oxygen therapy by nasal cannulae, as well as better quality of life by producing significant, subjective reduction of dyspnea, olfactory sensation, oral intake, weight gain and an increase in the overall sense of wellbeing because of aesthetic factors, feeling of independence and a trend towards less depression and improved morale.

An interesting extension of Heimlich's original method of delivering transtracheal oxygen is the method to deliver oxygen directly to the trachea via a small-bore catheter (Denver Hospital, USA). Regular cleaning of this catheter will ensure its proper function; in fact, cleaning twice daily with warm running water and a few drops of antibacterial soap is recommended. Then the catheter should be dried with a clean paper towel and allowed to air dry [10].

Another system for administering oxygen transtracheally is a permanently implanted polymer oxygen tube, that is placed subcutaneously from a tracheal insertion point to a skin exit site that is usually in a convenient area beneath the breast (Swedish Hospital Medical Center, Seattle).

This approach allows the user to completely hide all evidence of the oxygen-administering catheter and associated oxygen-delivery tubing. This oxygen catheter placement is an interesting technique and will be more widely available in the near future.

Transtracheal oxygen therapy is not a procedure without complications. However, these are relatively less severe and rare in comparison to the potential benefits (Table 4) [10].

Table 4. Benefits and complications of TTOT

Benefits	Complications
• Significant reduction in oxygen flow rate in comparison to nasal cannulae • No nasal, face or ear irritation or soreness • No dry effects on the nasal and oropharyngeal mucosa • Increase of patient outdoor activities due to longer lasting oxygen	• Inadvertent catheter dislodgement • Mild transient increase in sputum production • Transient dryness • Minor bleeding at site and time of insertion • Subcutaneous emphysema in head and neck region

Oxygen Economizers

Oxygen economizers are devices that, at the same flow, allow a greater amount of FiO_2; they are useful in terms of savings and in case of the need for high oxygen flow.

Different types are available on the market. They can divided into the following two groups:

1. Continuous flow economizers: oxymizer and pendant
2. Intermittent flow economizers: pulse system, demand system, hybrid [11].

The reservoir is a little container (about 20 cc) interposed on the length of the oxygen delivery tube, that swells during expiration and deflates during inspiration, in this way increasing the quantity of oxygen inhaled at every breath [11]. This resevoir operates by storing oxygen in a small chamber during exhalation for subsequent delivery during early-phase inhalation and it is driven by the patient's nasal inspiratory and expiratory pressures. Two models of continuous flow economizers are available: the **oxymizer** and the **pendant**.

The delivery efficiencies of the two are roughly equivalent. Compared with continuous flow oxygen, reservoir cannulae are two to four times as efficacious. They reduce oxygen usage by lowering oxygen flow setting from 25 to 50% of that required for continuous flow oxygen to achieve equivalent SaO_2. The advantages of reservoir cannulae lie in their simplicity, reliability and low cost. The disadvantage is that they are larger and more noticeable than demand devices.

Pulse systems deliver oxygen early during inspiratory effort, giving more oxygen in the effective portion of the breath so that more oxygen is delivered to the alveoli. Timing affects pulse systems, but they do not appear to be affected by dilution because of the early delivery of oxygen during inspiration [11].

Demand flow is delivered through the entire inspiratory section of the breath. Demand system flow rates are not as high as with pulse systems, so the volume of oxygen delivered per breath to the alveoli is less. They are affected by timing and dilution [1].

Hybrid systems deliver oxygen in an intermediate way compared to the above devices.

In spite of their characteristics and their safeness and ease of use, reservoirs have not become popular in Italy [1]. The use of intermittent flow economizers is lower than that of continuous flow economizers, whose development has been promoted in the USA due to the high costs of oxygen transport and the reimbursement system to supplying industries [1].

Oxygen Devices for Tracheostomy

These devices must be placed at the open end of the endotracheal tube or on tracheostomy cannulae. Normal efficiency is reached after a few breaths. They are very simple to insert and to take out. They can be used by the patient himself or by a trained care giver.

They are disposable and they can't be sterilized or reused because of higher risk of infection (Fig. 7).

They must be changed every 24 hours to avoid accumulation of mucous and an increase of airway resistance. Shelf life is five years when properly stored in the

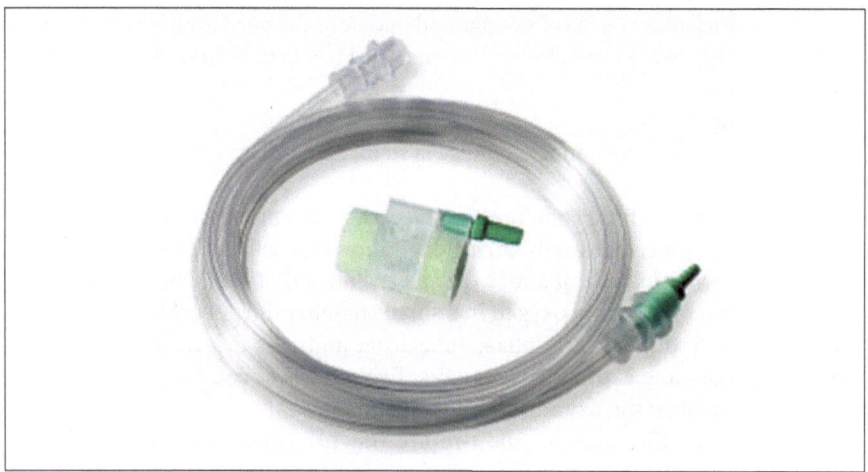

Fig. 7. Oxygen device for tracheostomy (Courtesy of Intersurgical, Wokingham, UK)

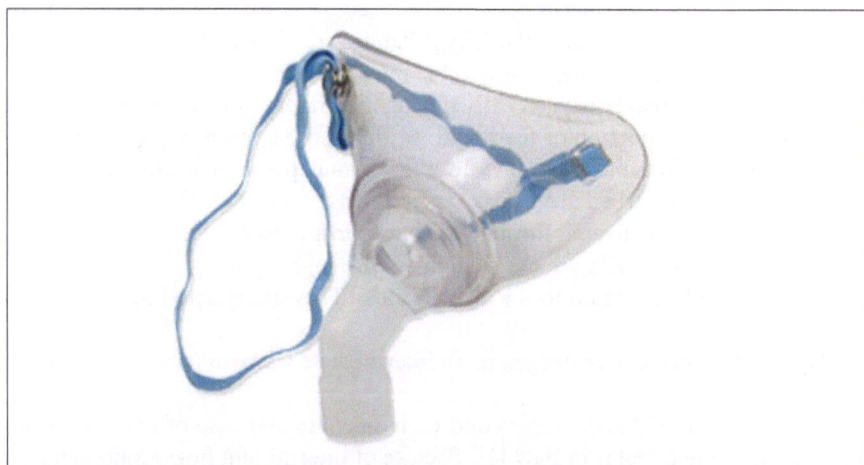

Fig. 8. Tracheostomy mask

sealed package.

They show an efficiency of humidification of inhaled air depending on tidal volume; for this reason the use in patients who have a tidal volume greater than the safe range (see table included in the device) must be evaluated very carefully.

In case the value of tidal volume is greater than recommended, the humidification of inhaled air is not sufficient, while in case of reduced tidal volume, the death space can cause carbon dioxide retention.

A good alternative choice is represented by tracheostomy masks (available in pediatric and adult sizes), supplied with a rubber band which is possible to fix on the patient's neck (Fig. 8). The interfaces on the market nowadays can be made of latex or can be latex-free. Patients affected by intolerance can choose the appropriate inhalation system.

In the end, oxygen, especially inhaled at medium to high flows, causes dryness of respiratory mucosa and sensations of "closed nose", sometimes inducing the patient to stop or to limit oxygen therapy.

With time, continuous dehydration causes the loss of epithelium and bleeding of mucosa.

In this case it is possible to use products with mechanical actions, composed of hyaluronic acid or carboxymethylglucan, in gel or liquid solutions (nasal sprays, nasal drops). These products allow lubrification, humidification and cleansing of nasal mucosa and renewal of local pH.

Acknowledgements. Figures 1, 3-6 and 8 are courtesy of Fiab SpA, Florence, Italy.

References

1. McCoy R (2000) Oxygen-conserving techniques and devices. Respir Care 45:95-104
2. Shapiro BA, Harrison RA, Walton JR (1994) Clinical application of blood gases, 3rd edn. Year Book Medical Publishers, Chicago, pp 169-179
3. Kacmarek R (2000) Delivery systems for long-term oxygen therapy. Respir Care 45:84-92
4. ATS Statement: Standards for the Diagnosis and Care of Patients with Chronic Obstructive Pulmonary Disease (1995) Am J Respir Crit Care Med 152(5 Pt 2): S77-S121
5. Bolliger CT, Mathur PN, Beamis JF, et al. (2002) ERS/ATS statement on interventional pulmonology. Eur Respir J 19:356-373
6. Orvidas LJ, Kasperbauer JL, Staats BA, Olsen KD (1998) Long-term clinical experience with transtracheal catheters. Mayo Clin Proc 73:739-744
7. Benditt J, Pollock M, Roa J, Celli B (1993) Transtracheal delivery of gas decreases the oxygen cost of breathing. Am Rev Respir Dis 147:1207-1210
8. Christopher KL, Spofford BT, Petrun MD, McCarty DC, Goodman JR, Petty TL (1987) A program for transtracheal oxygen delivery: assessment of safety and efficacy. Ann Intern Med 107:802-808
9. Wesmiller SW, Hoffman LA, Sciurba FC, Ferson PF, Johnson JT, Dauber JH (1990) Exercise tolerance during nasal cannula and transtracheal oxygen delivery. Am Rev Respir Dis 141:789-791
10. Lucas J (1988) Selecting the optimal oxygen system. In: Lucas J, Golish JA (eds) Home respiratory care. Appleton & Lange, Norwalk, pp 59-94
11. Murgia A, Scano G, Palange P, et al. (2004) Linee guida per la ossigenoterapia a lungo termine (OTLT). Aggiornamento anno 2004. Rass Pat App Resp 19:206-219

Telemedicine and LTOT in Italy: a 20-Year Experience

R. W. Dal Negro, P. Turco

As reported in the second chapter of this book, the difficulties of effectively managing and monitoring ever-growing numbers of patients distributed over large territories stimulated specialists who were involved in long-term oxygen treatment (LTOT) programs to radically change their approach to the chronic management of patients with severe respiratory disease needing continuous oxygen at home.

Although it is praiseworthy, the model for intervention used and consolidated in Italy (i.e., a model based for several years on small numbers of health professionals – doctors and nurses – and on groups of volunteers periodically aiding patients at home in their daily activities) frequently proved to be inadequate in ensuring the strict monitoring that is needed for the great majority of these patients. Moreover, although irreplaceable, the involvement of local volunteers (and of new organizations) who frequently took on institutional roles led paradoxically to the partial unawareness of health institutions of the real burden of LTOT, which was generally neglected or underestimated in their public health planning documents.

From a general point of view, economic resources for public health progressively decreased in those years (such as at the end of the 1980s), while the regulatory approach to LTOT remained lax or nonexistent throughout Italy. Depending on both the local sensitivity to the problem and the personal engagement of doctors and nurses, the net result was the spontaneous development of a large number of uncontrolled and heterogeneous protocols for managing LTOT around Italy. The total economic impact and the true cost-effectiveness of these local protocols were unknown and were not assessed at that time.

In order to minimize or reduce the effects of these variables, our group moved toward innovative technologies that were aimed at daily telemetric contacts with patients at home and their interactive remote monitoring. We were (and still are) convinced that telemedicine should provide, even though remote, the advantages of a specialist organization, of equipment, and of a particular know-how that can be available at the patient's home when needed.

The project started with the triennial support (1990-1992) of the Department for Public Health of the Regione Veneto (project no. 324/03/90), who strongly supported this pioneer research (Fig. 1) with the aim of providing patients and their families with new health and therapeutic options able to encourage de-hospitalization while greatly improving quality of life at home. The project was also carried out with the support of the National Research Council (CNR, document no. 6345/91) and of VitalAire Italia, who agreed to carry out technological research and development according to our ideas and suggestions.

This pioneer system for daily telemetric home monitoring of LTOT patients was launched in 1991, and was founded on the use of liquid oxygen. Liquid oxygen was preferred to other systems because it was assessed as the most convenient from the perspective of patients (e.g., in terms of quality of oxygen delivered; environmental noise; personal costs due to long-term power use; patients' autonomy and mobilization) and of institutions (e.g., the health opportunity delivered to LTOT patients and their families; health and social costs).

In the beginning, the telemetric system consisted of one central unit (CU) and of several peripheral units (PUs) for data collection, which were located at patients' homes: this domiciliary equipment was very practical and did not require a high level of skill and training for patients and their care-givers [1-3]. All

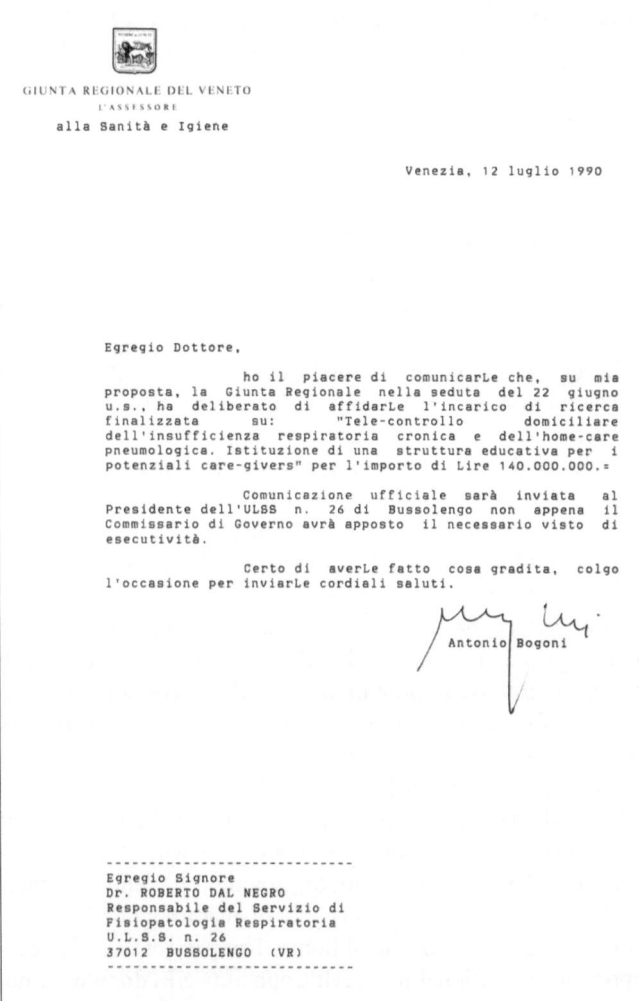

Fig. 1. The first document issued by the Department of Public Health in 1990 concerning the domiciliary tele-monitoring of patients needing LTOT. This document initiated the course of respiratory telemedicine in Italy

patients connected to the CU several times a day, and vital signs and functional indicators were easily collected according to the particular protocol scheduled by specialist staff for each patient, depending on their original disease and severity. In other words, each patient had scheduled timing (frequency and duration) for connection over 24 hours. Moreover, under specific conditions, such as in the case of particularly unstable patients with a rapidly changing clinical status, operators had the opportunity to activate further connections in order to check these patients more closely. When needed, patients could make further spontaneous connections to the CU directly. Furthermore, patients at home could transmit a priority message to the specialist group and call for immediate intervention (SOS) by pushing a red button that was easily visible on top of the domiciliary equipment. Once received, the priority message was switched into both visual and acoustic signals that remained active until released by the CU operator(s).

The first set-up of the system is shown in Fig. 2. At that time, the CU consisted of a PC 386 (4 MB RAM and 80 MB hard disk) including a VGA monochromatic monitor, a keyboard, a serial printer (80 columns), and a serial asynchronous modem for domiciliary connections to each PU. The UNIX operating system was chosen because it is a standard "multi-tasking" system allowing operators to carry out simultaneous operations in real time.

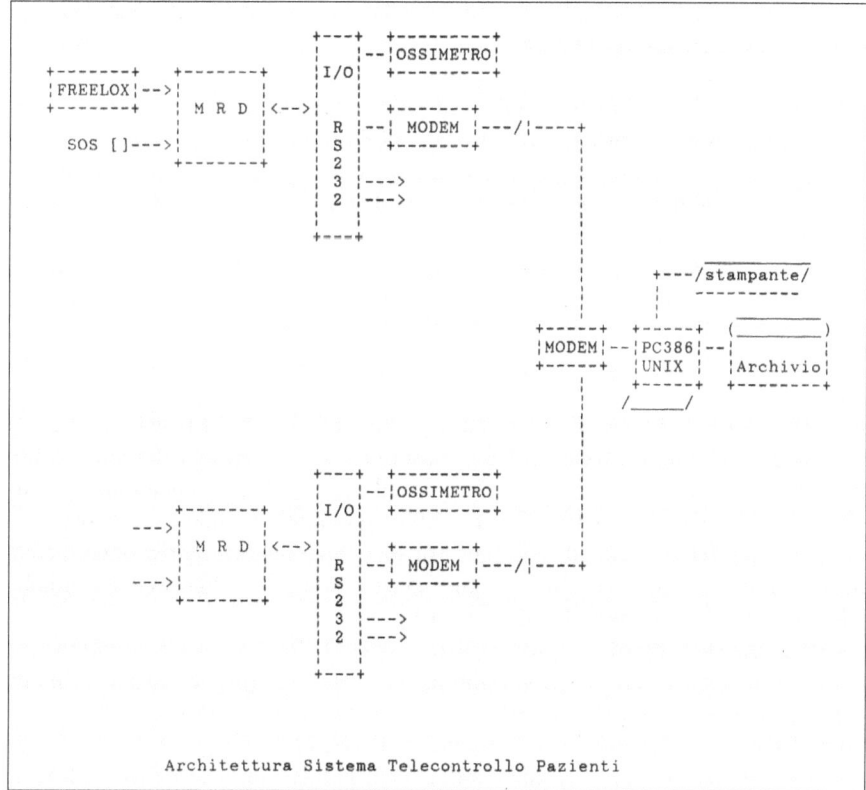

Fig. 2. Set-up of the first version of the telemetric system

The application software basically consisted of:

A - Operator functions:
- PU initialization
- Patient's personal history database management
- Patient's display and printing cards
- Chronological analysis of alarm signals
- Management of current alarm messages
- System shut-down

B - Automatic functions:
- Periodic PU scanning
- Acquisition and storage of patient's current data
- Management of alarm messages
- System diagnostics

Each PU consisted of a microprocessor, a few analog lines with an analog/digital converter, a few digital lines, a series of four RS232 serial asynchronous lines, and one serial asynchronous modem. A pushbutton was also included on the domiciliary equipment.

The software (firmware) included both peripheral functions and functions for data and message communication to the CU. The automatic PU diagnostic system was also in continuous operation.

According to this configuration, the local peripheral connections to the PU were:
- A pulse-oxymeter (for the noninvasive measurement and monitoring of oxygen saturation and of heart frequency - minimum recording 5 min)
- A liquid oxygen container, which was modified to allow both the acquisition and the storage of data in terms of calculation of O_2 consumption and O_2 reserve.

In the first version of the system, collectable data were: heart frequency (HF), O_2 saturation, O_2 consumption, and O_2 reserve in the container for liquid oxygen, the structure of which was modified for this project (Freelox) (Fig. 3A-C).

Furthermore, by automatically comparing the theoretical trend (hours) of 90% Freelox emptying (which can be calculated by knowing the total O_2 content in the Freelox and the medical O_2 prescription/day - l/min/day) with the true trend (hours) of oxygen emptying (i.e., the time for consuming 90% O_2, which depends on the patient's true adherence to the O_2 prescription/day), we obtained a quantitative indicator of the patient's compliance to the LTOT program. O_2 under-use or over-use became easily detectable, their causes investigated, and timely preventive or corrective measures could be taken. In this configuration, the domiciliary PUs were extendible, with up to 100 PUs connected to the same CU.

Since the start-up of the project of telemetric LTOT, particular attention was paid by doctors and nurses to the training of patients and their care-givers (in our experience, 95% were patients' relatives) in managing these technical devices at home. Their activities and the corresponding outcomes are reported in other chapters of this book. Despite specialists' initial fears, patients (and care-givers) did not show any apprehension in taking a new approach to their disease: they immediate-

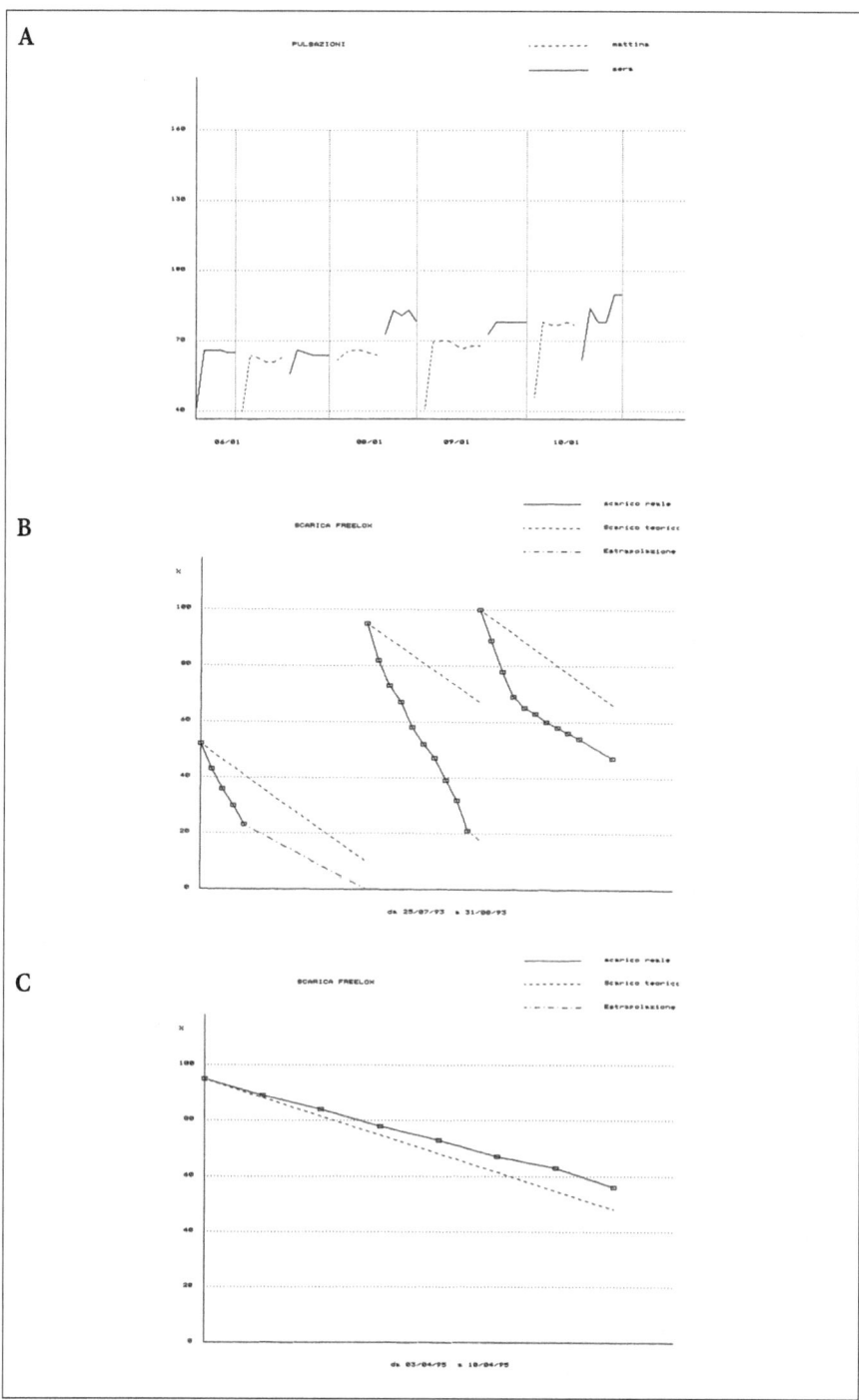

Fig. 3. Examples of original data acquisition from LTOT patients managed at home via the telemetric system. A Heart rate monitoring during the morning (- - -) and at night (——). B, C The trend of Freelox emptying in a non-compliant and in a compliant LTOT patient, respectively

ly cooperated to the best of their abilities. Both their skill and their motivation proved to be totally independent of their original cultural and social levels.

In a short time, the telemetric system led to a substantial drop in home visits to LTOT subjects. These home visits were carried out periodically to check all patients independent of their condition (stable or unstable), without any possibility of concentrating medical efforts only on those cases truly needing specialist intervention. Frequently, these visits were a sort of "social need" for the patient and a "social duty" for the doctor, without any intrinsic value for the parties involved. Spot visits, carried out, for example, once a week or twice a month, were, and still are in our opinion, inadequate for monitoring these subjects, because of severe chronic respiratory condition that could suddenly deteriorate dramatically. In these cases, only quick recognition of the problem and prompt medical intervention were (and still are) the true key issues.

Furthermore, under certain operational conditions (e.g., too many subjects to check, too wide territories to monitor, logistic and geographical difficulties to manage, etc.) the possibilities of effective daily personal contact with all LTOT patients diminish, and any organization based on such a "staff-dependent" working model proves inadequate in the short term.

With telemetric monitoring, once any dangerous domiciliary event is detected by the CU operator, or once a patient's SOS signal is received automatically activating a direct telephone check, ambulance is sent immediately from the hospital to the patient's house. In other words, home medical intervention is focused only on severe events or emergency calls, with all daily routine activities managed via telemetric contacts with LTOT patients (and care-givers). Moreover, all data from PUs (such as extra calls, SOS calls, instrumental diagnostics) were registered for each patient in the CU, constituting personal histories of all patients, which could be used for consultation and/or statistical analysis.

As mentioned before, all patients admitted to the LTOT program of telemetric home management received specific educational support by the staff of nurses who had been specifically instructed to achieve the maximal compliance and adherence to the project from patients. Before including a new LTOT patient, nurses had to explain the new LTOT protocol of intervention, to investigate the patient's social condition and familial setting, and to confirm their true motivation and agreement with the telemetric LTOT activities. After this initial investigational phase, nurses passed to the specific educational phase of the patient and their care-giver(s): a type of school dedicated to chronic respiratory failure education based on open discussion, slide presentations, video shows, and practicing with the domiciliary devices by simulating emergency events (e.g., which clinical signs to evaluate before sending the SOS message, quick use of the red SOS button, how to contact the CU operator, etc.).

While doctors had to decide and prescribe the daily medical strategy of home treatment, nurses had to explain the correct use of drugs and deliver the "home pharmacy" for the next 4-week period to patients, to keep the accounts, and to check and report the patients' compliance to treatments.

Moreover, nurses also had to check the patients' and their care-givers' suggestions periodically by means of questionnaires: following data collection and data processing, their reports were used for discussion during the activities of the "self-help groups" and for the continuous improvement and optimization of LTOT management. In agreement with the literature [4], this ongoing educational and motivational support produced important results.

Within a couple of years, LTOT management benefited substantially from the use of the telemetric approach: the very promising results of this new approach also contributed to the decision by the Regional Public Health Department to institute the "domiciliary hospitalization" for LTOT patients (see chapter 2). As in the case of a regular in-patient, those LTOT subjects who were telemetrically monitored at home were managed by the hospital medical staff of lung specialists, who contacted them daily at home, checked their vital signs via computer, and updated their oxygen and pharmacological needs. Furthermore, all patients were also visited at home, and arterial gas analysis was performed every 2-3 months to evaluate their general conditions and vital parameters. In 2004, the ATS/ERS joint document reported a protocol for the management of LTOT patients, which was very similar to this one, also in terms of timing for arterial blood gas checks and specialist visits [5].

The second release of this system was made 3-4 years later. The most relevant changes were: further peripheral connections, and particularly connections with the mechanical ventilator; on-line diagnostics of peripheral equipment; management of the patients' quality-of-life questionnaires; improvement and extension of the graphics package (which allows display in real time of the patients' parametrical time-course); implementation of a statistics package; installation of a second parallel modem to ensure the immediate and independent acquisition of SOS messages (Fig. 4).

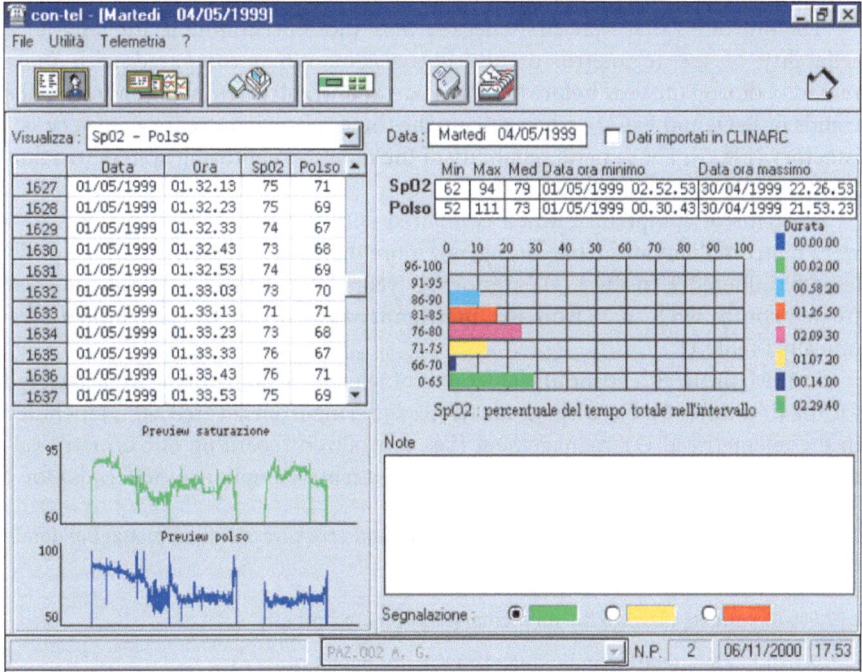

Fig. 4. Example of data acquisition with the second version of the telemetric system; in particular, O_2 saturation and heart rate

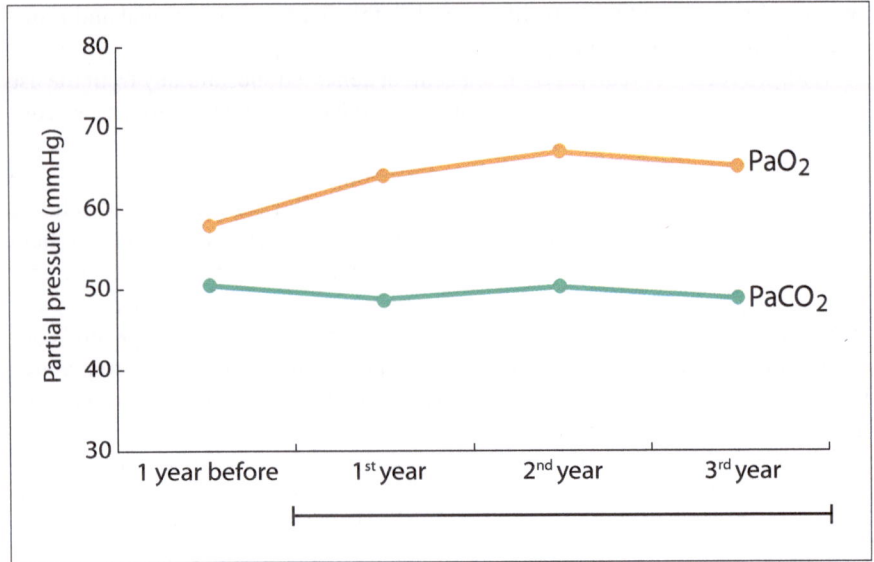

Fig. 5. PaO$_2$ and PaCO$_2$ time-course carried out 1 year before patient inclusion in the telemetric LTOT program and during the next 3 years (n=141)

Moreover, the new release was also oriented to the organization of several CUs connected to communicate with each other in order to create the first national database for patients in home LTOT.

The outcomes that were first checked were those pertaining to the long-term reliability of the telemetric monitoring system. When compared with those recorded during the year before the inclusion of telemetric remote monitoring, the trends of PaO$_2$ and PaCO$_2$ values during the three subsequent years were very satisfactory (Fig. 5). The general reliability of the remote monitoring system was thus further confirmed and highlighted.

In terms of compliance, when compared with the 10%-15% of patients who were noncompliant at the beginning, not more than 1% of patients claimed problems of adherence to the LTOT protocol 3 years later. This crucial outcome was further confirmed by data from the questionnaires answered by each patient periodically (Table 1).

In 1994, the health economic outcomes of telemetric home LTOT were assessed for the first time [6]. For 61 patients (n=52 suffering from severe COPD) included in the telemetric LTOT management (i.e., centralized recording of oxymetry values, heart rate, O$_2$ consumption, O$_2$ reserve, patients' compliance, SOS calls) for 2

Table 1. Results of the periodic check of patients' and care-givers' skill in managing domiciliary devices for telemetric LTOT

- 72.9% of patients manage the domiciliary equipment properly
- 96.7% of home-attending individuals use the equipment properly
- 91.6% use the red emergency alarm button properly

years, the number of hospital admissions and their duration (days) were calculated and compared yearly with those of a corresponding pre-telemetric period of 12 months. Both direct and indirect costs were calculated in US dollars, indirect costs being calculated only for the seven still-working subjects. Hospital admissions and duration of hospitalization decreased significantly (from 1.8/year to 0.5/year and from 36.9 days/year to 7.4 days/year, respectively). Direct costs dropped from US $ 769 000 to 125 300, while indirect costs (such as job dependency in the seven working subjects) dropped from US $ 51 800 to 11 700 in the same period (Figs. 6, 7). These data were also confirmed in other reports several years later [7].

As confirmed by recent studies [8], significant improvements in patients' quality of life were obtained with LTOT and further contributed toward both the economic and the social convenience and utility of this particular domiciliary treatment.

Recently, the tele-home monitoring of LTOT patients has been adopted by other groups, who confirmed the same trend of utility of the program for both the

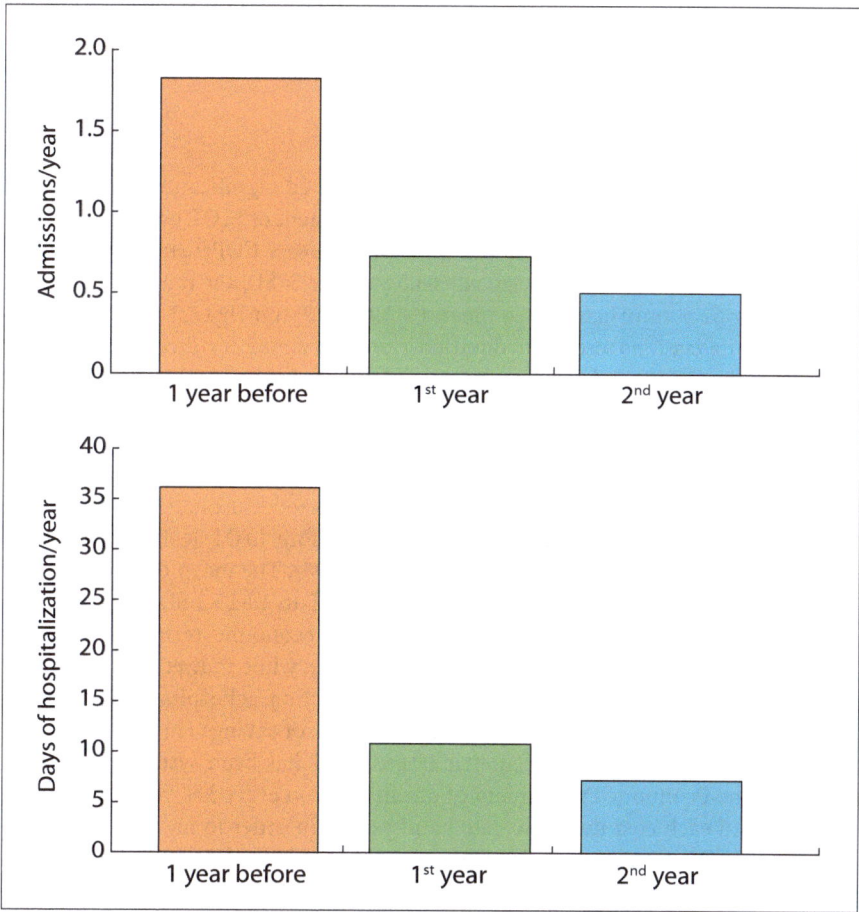

Fig. 6. Health economic outcomes from a 3-year period (1 year before and 2 years after telemetric LTOT): changes in hospital admissions and duration/patient/year

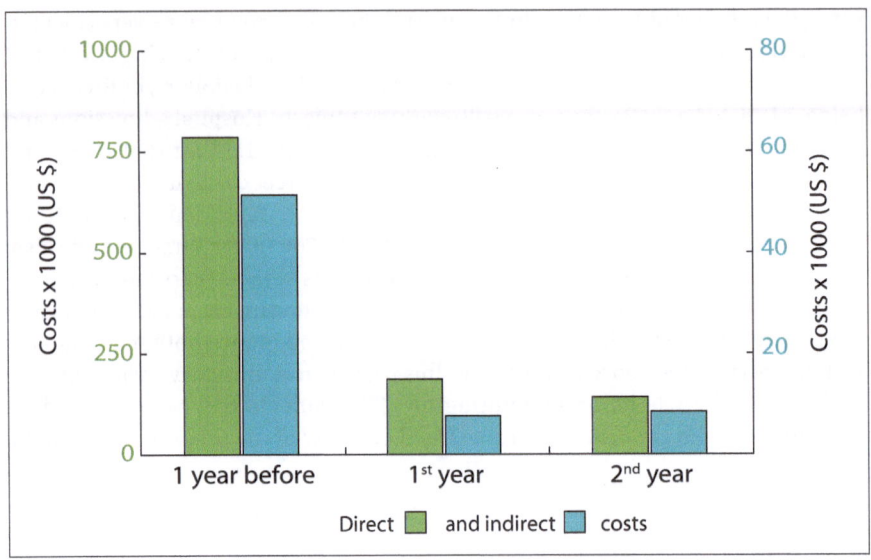

Fig. 7. Health economic outcomes from a 3-year period (1 year before and 2 years after telemetric LTOT): direct and indirect costs/patient/year

patients and the community [9].

The frequency of lower airway infection dropped significantly during the 2 years of tele-home monitoring and remote management of LTOT patients. The first survey was initially carried out in a sample of 82 severe COPD subjects regularly managed at home (62 males; mean age 63.5 years±8.5 SD, age range 47-74 years; mean PaO_2=62.3 mmHg±3.8 SD; mean $PaCO_2$=46.7 mmHg±4.2 SD). The number of hospitalizations and their duration were calculated for each subject in the year preceding LTOT and for 2 years after inclusion in the LTOT tele-monitoring program. Infectious events registered amounted to 22 during the pre-LTOT year; 8 during the first and during the second year of tele-home LTOT. Due to the occurrence of a lung infection, mean PaO_2 dropped to 52.1 mmHg±5.5 SD, and $PaCO_2$ to 53.3 mmHg±4.6 SD, but no fatal event was registered. Hospitalizations changed from a mean value of 0.3/patient/year±0.5 SD before LTOT to 0.1±0.3 SD and 0.0±0.3 SD in the following 2 years (Anova, p<0.005). The mean duration of hospitalization dropped from 4.9±10.3 SD before LTOT to 1.5±5.2 SD and 1.1±3.7 in the following 2 years (Anova, p<0.005) [10]. In economic terms, direct costs dropped from US $ 12 600 to 2 100 per patient/year, while indirect costs dropped from US $ 7 400 to 1 730 per patient/year, the reduction in hospitalizations and in pharmacological expenditure being the main causes of savings [11].

The health economics of telemetric home LTOT has been systematically controlled by the Economic Department of our institution every 3-4 years (from 1995 to 2004), and each cost item calculated and valued in order to monitor the evolution of the LTOT costs/patient/day. Changes recorded in the last decade are reported in Table 2. In general terms, it is possible to affirm that the costs per patient for 1 year of continuous and effective home telemetric LTOT are lower than those of a single hospitalization for COPD exacerbation: there are substantial total savings for

Table 2. Analytical costs/patient/day of telemetric LTOT in the last decade (€)

	1995*	1998	2002	2004
Gas analysis (+ other procedures)	0.62	1.39	1.60	1.64
O_2 (1.5 l/min x 18 h/day)	6.66	7.90	7.90	7.39
Medical staff (visits, medical reports, etc.)	0.83	0.97	1.06	1.18
Nurses (database management, drug distribution, etc.)	1.03	1.14	1.09	1.12
Pharmaceutical costs	0.64	0.83	1.08	1.05
Telemedicine network	0.21	0.31	0.39	0.41
General costs	0.57	0.91	1.01	1.32
Physiokinesitherapy (PKT) + vent. nursing	-	-	0.68**	2.70***
Total costs	10.56	13.45	14.13	16.81

* From [9]; **Costs due to only PKT; *** Costs due to PKT plus specific nursing for the domiciliary ventilator

the community and quality of life is much improved for patients and their families.

A further crucial point when evaluating the LTOT outcomes of long-term patients is to assess their survival. A couple of decades ago the mean survival of LTOT patients who had PaO_2 values persistently lower than 60 mmHg was 20%-40% in the third year of LTOT [12] (Fig. 8).

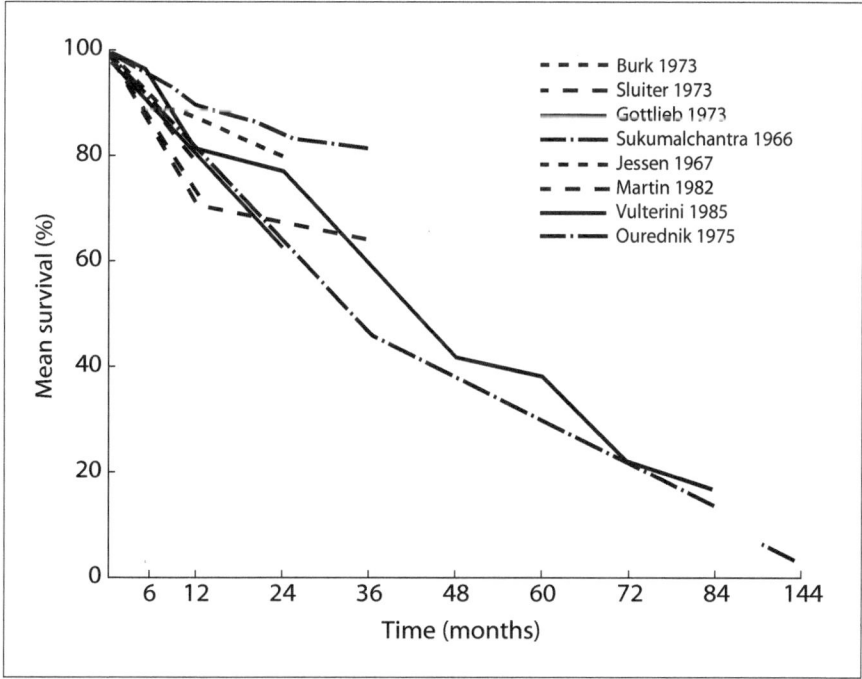

Fig. 8. Mean survival as observed in different studies carried out on LTOT patients between 1966 and 1985

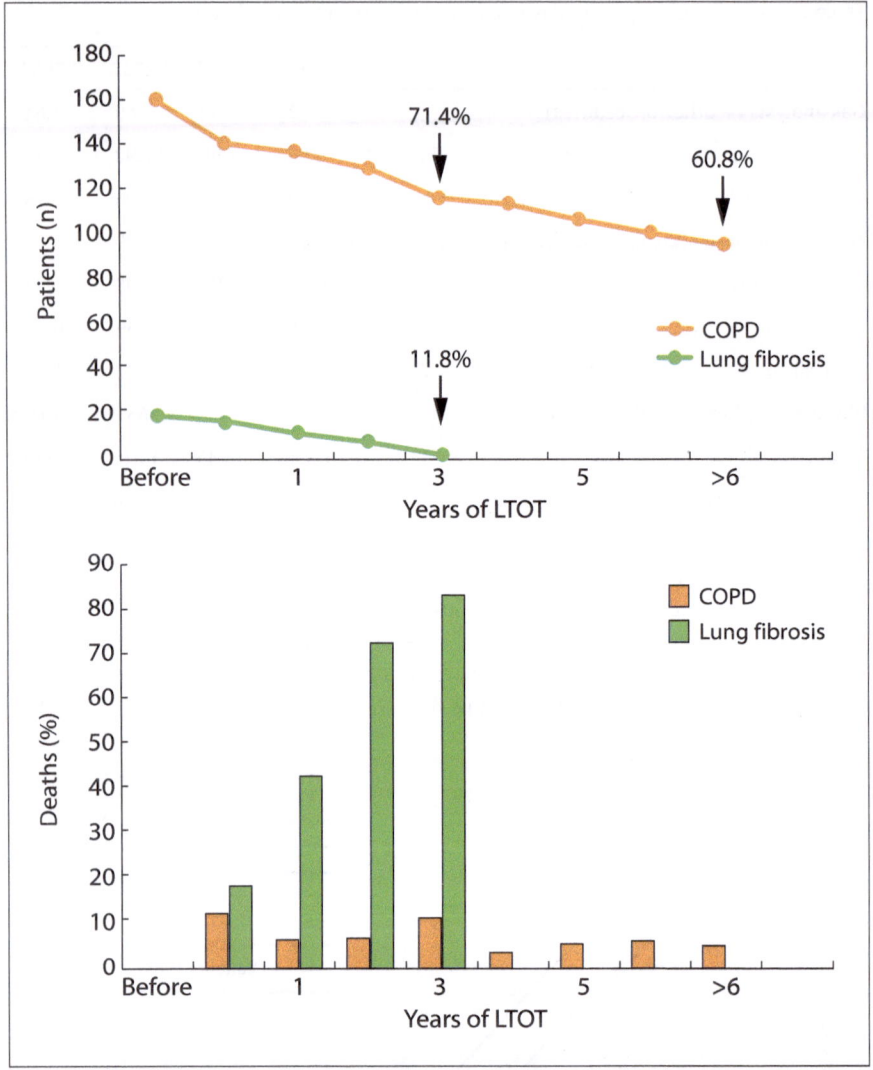

Fig. 9. Mean survival observed in tele-monitored LTOT patients in 2004 (n=165). Different long-term results were obtained in COPD and in fibrotic patients included in the tele-monitored LTOT program

In 2004, the mean survival was calculated in a sample (n=165) of tele-monitored LTOT patients directly from the database of our institution: 71.4% of severe COPD patients were alive after 3 years, and 60.8% were still alive after more than 6 years – a good result when compared with that obtained in the past according to the traditional approach of LTOT management (Fig. 9).

All these data, which are mainly derived from severe COPD patients, have been periodically confirmed in our 20-year experience and also by other groups [4]. However, a recent paper concerning an Australian group's experience with LTOT showed conflicting results in terms of survival, although the causes of these poor results were not explained by the authors [13].

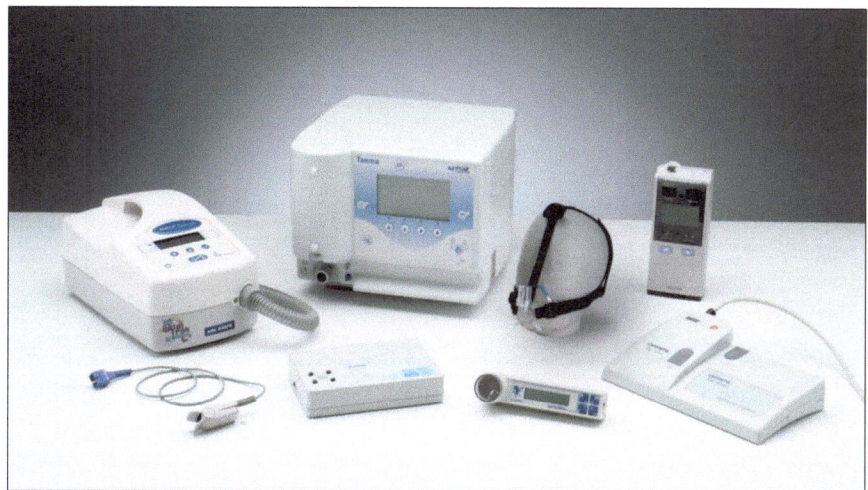

Fig. 10. All the devices now available in the most recent version of the domiciliary telemetric system for monitoring LTOT patients: different modules can be combined according to the patient's needs (Courtesy of VitalAire Italia SpA, Milan, Italy)

In agreement with the literature [14, 15], the mean survival of patients proved substantially lower in the presence of lung fibrosis, with only 11.8% of fibrotic patients alive after 3 years of LTOT (Fig. 9).

The different causes of fatal events were also investigated anatomically in the majority of deaths: pulmonary embolism and acute heart failure were the most common in COPD patients (58.8% and 14.8%, respectively), pneumonia being the least common (2.9%). A condition corresponding to "end-stage lung" was the only cause of death within our group of patients with lung fibrosis.

Unlike the old versions, which mainly consisted of an "ad hoc" system for a single pathology, the most recent version of the telemetric system (i.e., the third release) was created to fit multiple pathologies to be managed at home, and comprises a modular system in which several parameters can be controlled in real time.

Recent PU additions include a spirometer, an ECG, a capnograph, and a ventilator, making the PU configuration much easier and more fitting to each patient's needs (Fig. 10). In the last version, both data collection and connections to and from the patient's home are much easier and have been further updated; the option to manage questionnaires by patients and/or doctors (or care-givers) is now operating; several parties involved in the management of LTOT patients can contribute actively according to their own role; all activities can be scheduled precisely; several parameters from different diagnostic equipment can be integrated immediately in order to assess the patient's condition more precisely and in real time (Fig. 11).

All technical improvements characterizing the last version of the telemetric facilities are described in chapter 7.

In conclusion, a long race has been run from the first approach to the long-term oxygen treatment of patients with chronic respiratory disease at home.

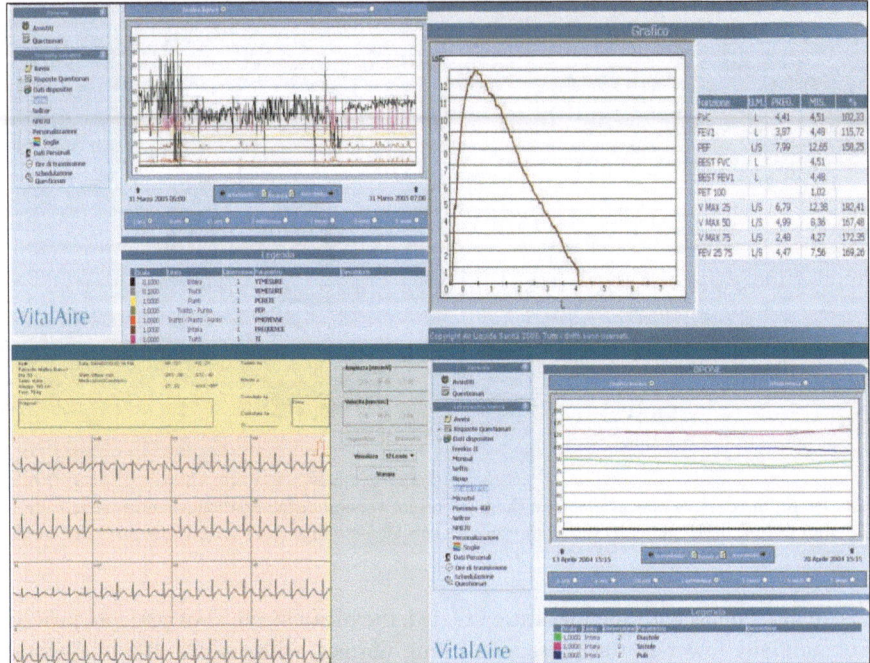

Fig. 11. Examples of multiple parametrical control during LTOT carried out with the last version of the telemetric system (Con-Tel II)

During the last 20 years, the general approach to LTOT has progressed from involving volunteers only, which represented the original positive boost, to the remote monitoring and centralized tele-management in real time that is currently available.

A few pioneer specialists and nurses trusting in an innovative and promising scientific vision, a few enlightened public health politicians who were "ahead of their own time", and a few creative engineers and technologists were responsible for the introduction and promotion of telemedicine in Italy in the last two decades. Their strong will and motivation, their compassion for patients with severe respiratory disease needing a continuous supply of oxygen at home, together with their great respect for patients' and families' troubles, were the unique ingredients which led them to "think different" several years ago and to arrive at the present opportunities for the effective remote management of LTOT patients at home.

References

1. Dal Negro R, Turco P, Pomari C (1991) Progetto di telemetria per l'home care respiratoria. Risultati preliminari. Rass Pat App Resp 6:111
2. Dal Negro R, Turco P, Pomari C (1992) A telemetric system for respiratory home care. 2nd International. Conference on Advances in Pneumology Rehabilitation and Management of Chronic Respiratory Failure. Venice, Proceedings, p 156
3. Refice G, Dal Negro R (1997) Assistenza sanitaria di qualità. Management e Telecomunicazioni. 12:37-40
4. Gibbons D, Conneelly J, Smith J (2002) An audit of provision of long-term oxygen therapy for

COPD patients. Prof Nurse 18:107-110
5. Celli BR, MacNee W (2004) Standards for the diagnosis and treatment of patients with COPD: a summary of the ATS/ERS positive paper. Eur Respir J 23:932-946
6. Micheletto C, Pomari C, Righetti P, Dal Negro R (1994) A 2-year health economics survey on 61 subjects in telemetric LTOT: preliminary results. Eur Respir J (Suppl 7)18:266
7. Ringbaek TJ, Viskum K, Lange P (2002) Does long-term oxygen therapy reduce hospitalization in hypoxemic chronic obstructive pulmonary disease? Eur Respir J 20:38-42
8. Eaton T, Lewis C, Young P, Kennedy Y, Garrett JE, Kolbe J (2004) Long-term oxygen therapy improves health-related quality of life. Respir Med 98:285-293
9. Maiolo C, Mohamed EI, Fiorani CM, De Lorenzo A (2003) Home telemonitoring for patients with severe respiratory illness: the Italian experience. J Telemed Telecare 9:67-71
10. Dal Negro R, Pomari C, Micheletto C (1995) Ossigenoterapia domiciliare a lungo termine (OTLT) sotto controllo telematico: aspetti farmacoeconomici. Farmacoeconomia 2:43-46
11. Micheletto C, Pomari C, Dal Negro R (1994) Infezioni acute delle basse vie respiratorie durante ossigenoterapia a lungo termine. 3rd International Meeting "Highlights in Pneumology", 25-26 March, Proceedings, p 75
12. Paramelle B, Brambilla C, Geraads A, Rigaud D (1984) Indications et critères de decision de l'oxygénothérapie de suppléance pour l'hypoxémie chronique. Rev Fran Mal Respir 22-37
13. Cranston JM, Nguyen AM, Crockett A (2004) The relative survival of COPD patients on long-term oxygen therapy in Australia: a comparative study. Respirology 9:237-242
14. Strom K, Boman G (1993) Long-term oxygen therapy in parenchymal lung diseases: an analysis of survival. The Swedish Society of Chest Medicine. Eur Respir J 6:1264-1270
15. Chailleux E, Fauroux B, Binet F, Dautzemberg B, Polu JM (1996) Predictor of survival in patients receiving domiciliary oxygen therapy or mechanical ventilation. Chest 108:741-749

New Telemonitoring Technologies in Italy

C. Guglielmetti, M. Gaiani

The ALS Con-Tel II system is a complex system that allows clinical monitoring in the home of the patient, and is comprised of two structural elements:
- **ALS Con-Tel II**: a home electromedical device.
- **ALS Gate**: a dedicated Web portal used to consult and assess captured clinical parameters.

ALS Con-Tel II

This is an active medical device which depends on a power source for operation, and is used either alone or in combination with other medical devices.

Its main feature is to provide physicians or healthcare professionals with all information concerning analysis, early diagnosis, monitoring or treatment of clinical conditions, health, diseases, or birth defects.

Certification

For medical devices, there are legislative provisions dictating that technologies should be designed, built, maintained and operated effectively, efficiently and – most of all – safely.

ALS Con-Tel II is built to the requirements of the laws and directives in force, and is provided with the EC051 mark (complete Quality Assurance System)(Fig. 1).

Reference Framework – System Standards
- UNI EN ISO 9001 (2000) Quality Management Systems – Requirements
- UNI CEI EN ISO 13485 (2002) Quality Management Systems – Special Requirements for Enforcement of UNI EN ISO 9001
- UNI EN ISO 9000 (2000) Quality Management Systems – Fundamentals and Terminology

Reference Framework – Product Standards
- EN 60601-1 General Safety Standards 12 - 1998
- CEI EN 60601-1-4 General Requirements - Programmable Electrical Medical Systems
- UNI EN 865 2000 Pulse Oxymeters - Special Requirements
- CEI EN 60601-1-2:1993 Medical Electrical Equipment – Part 1 General Safety Requirements 2 – Collateral Standard: Electromagnetic Compatibility-Requirements and Testing
- CEI EN 60601-1-2:2001 Medical Electrical Equipment – Part 1-2 General Safety

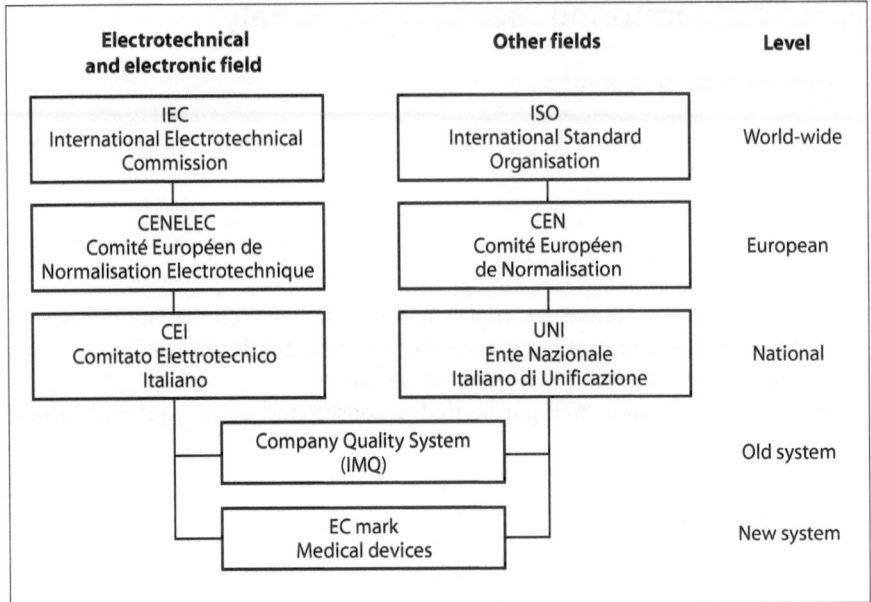

Fig. 1. Company Quality System requirements for manufacture and control

Requirements Collateral Standard: Electromagnetic Compatibility-Requirements and Testing
- UNI CEI EN ISO 14971 Application of Risk Management to Medical Devices
- EN 980 Graphical Symbols for Use in the Labelling of Medical Devices
- EN 1041 Information Supplied by the Manufacturer with Medical Devices

Reference Framework – Laws
- 93/42/EEC Council Directive concerning Medical Devices. Council of European Communities
- 89/336 EEC Electromagnetic Compatibility
- Legislative Decree No. 46 dated 24.02.1997 Implementation of Council Directive No. 93/42/EEC dated 14th June 1993 concerning Medical Devices
- Presidential Decree No. 224 dated 24.05.1988 Liability for Damages Due to Defective Products
- Legislative Decree No. 115 dated 17/3/1995 General Product Safety

The risk analysis for this device was performed according to the criteria as set forth in Standard EN 14971.

Because of its characteristics, "it is not a life-saving device, and it may not be used for emergency".

Features

ALS Con-Tel II is a modular medical device which makes it possible to quantitatively and non-invasively assess oxygen saturation in arterial haemoglobin. It also has additional features which make it able to capture and store instrumental parameters from medical devices and external sensors.

The input data from external devices and the data captured by the integrated oxymeter card are not processed before they are saved on the hard disk. Clinical parameters are captured by EC-marked devices through a protocol supplied by the manufacturer.

Through its simple and user-friendly graphics interface which can be managed entirely from the touch-screen monitor, ALS Con-Tel II has a number of additional features enabling:

- transfer of stored information to a dedicated Web portal through either a PSTN line or a LAN – either by means of an automatic process or on demand
- exchange of subsequent clinical information, such as notices and answers to customised questionnaires
- multilingual modes (Italian, English, French, Spanish, German)
- scheduled events, as indicated by a diary and a notice advising the patient that the deadline for acquisitions is approaching.

Security

Software securities make sure that:

- the data to be transmitted are correct
- the data retrieved from memory upon sending are actually the desired ones
- the system will not crash, because it can manage errors in the input fields completed by the user
- selection by touching the corresponding area in the screen with a finger is unequivocally identifiable by means of colours that are in contrast with the background
- a number of menus, which are accessible from a password-protected window, allow the installer to have access to serial port configuration features, assigning one of the listed devices to each of them.

The software is protected by routines which prevent any human or hardware input errors from causing a crash in the system, that would make the medical device unserviceable.

The operating system makes it possible to detect and therefore handle any hardware failures with messages and warnings; connection errors are possible, although serial ports are marked by numbers identifying them unequivocally.

Any voltage drops due to events resulting in the device suddenly switching off will cause no damage. The device will restart automatically. Once voltage has been restored and the device has been restarted, failed or incomplete data sent to the dedicated Web portal will be automatically restarted, and open tasks will be completed.

Technical Characteristics (Fig. 2)

Data Transmission
- By telephone (PSTN): 56K Modem
- By LAN (Local Area Network): RJ45 Ethernet connector (10/100 Ethernet card)

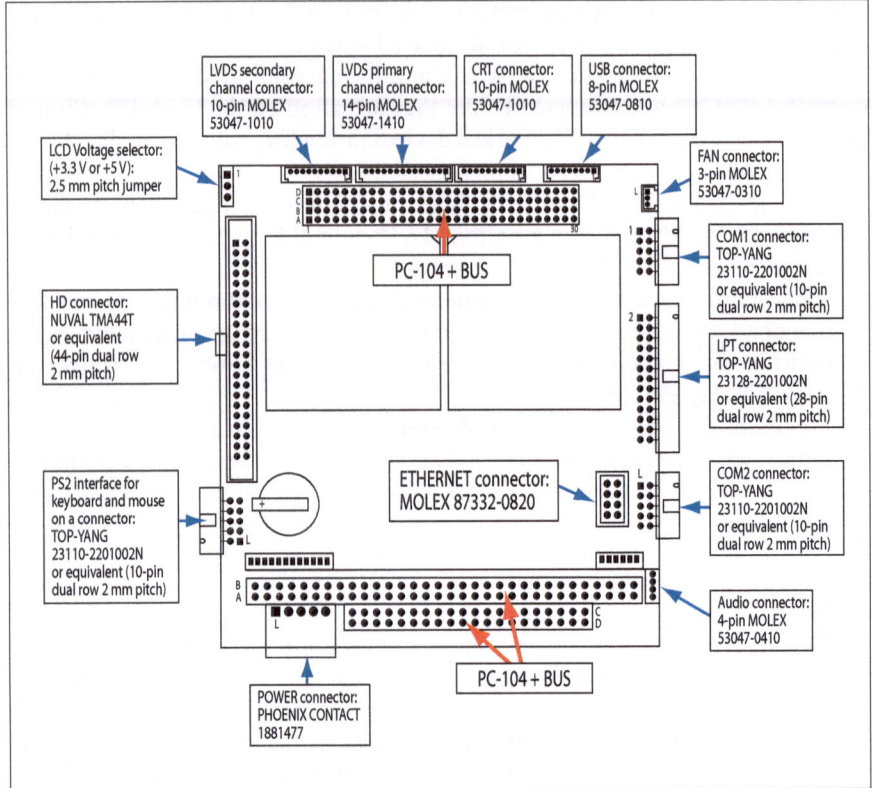

Fig. 2. Motherboard technical characteristics

Connection of External Medical Devices
- No. 4 RS 232 female serial ports
- No. 2 USB 1.1 ports
- No. 1 dedicated pulse oxymeter sensor port
- No. 1 PS2/external keyboard connector

Motherboard
- PC 104 card, VIA Eden ESP 700D 733 MhZ CPU

Mass Storage
- 2.5" 20 Gbyte HDD
- 128 Mbyte RAM
- 512 Kbyte ROM

Type of Monitor
- Touch-screen monitor – TFT 10.4" backlighted LCD – graphic resolution from 640 x 480 to 1024 x 768

Operating System
- Totally preinstalled and configured embedded XP

Application Software
- Developed under Visual Basic 6 (Microsoft environment) with fully visual interface design features and event-driven language

Output Data Format
- The connection between the device and the dedicated Web portal is through a SOAP connection (XML format) over TCP-IP

ALS Gate

This is a dedicated Web portal which was developed using new Microsoft technology that made it possible to create a very customisable application, which could not have been easily developed using traditional technologies.

The main core of the application is a totally configurable information management system. The system makes it possible to define the characteristics of each individual piece of information, and how it shall be displayed. All modules in the application rely on this core to organise the information to be managed.

Since this is a Web application, it ensures accessibility to users who are spread throughout the territory, as well as access through multiple platforms (PCs, PocketPCs, UMTS, etc.) (Fig. 3).

Security

As the application runs in a Web environment, security is ensured by the 128-bit SSL encryption protocol. All Internet communications between client and server travel

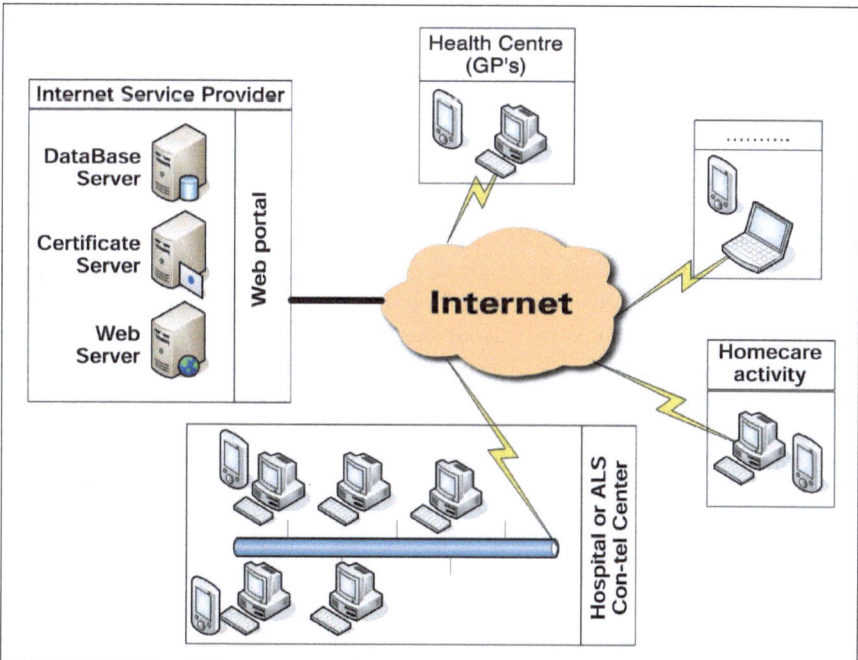

Fig. 3. The ALS Gate system

over a HTTPS (HyperText Transfer Protocol over Secure Socket Layer) protocol, which is a secure version of the HTTP protocol that is commonly adopted for Internet browsing.

In order to better understand this significant factor – i.e., security – for management of clinical parameters, it is important to correctly divide application security from infrastructural security.

Application Security

Application security was planned and implemented in the analysis and development phases in order to ensure integrity and protection of treated data.

Each user is assigned a pair of personal identification numbers:
- a Login code
- a Password code

These codes are generated through algorithms ensuring that they are unique and unrepeatable for all health care facilities.

Each examination is unequivocally matched by the personal identification numbers of the user who owns the data, and stored in daily files. For security reasons, the application receiving requests to send examinations (Web server) is resident on an appropriate server, which is separate from the server managing report filing.

Encrypted daily files containing reports are stored in a Data server rather than the Web server, in different folders. Encryption of daily files is maintained throughout the filing period.

Examinations are displayed through a browser using the SSL protocol, which integrates symmetrical private-key encryption.

Infrastructural Security

As far as infrastructural security is concerned, all possible hardware and software measures were taken to ensure continuous service provision and protection from attacks by ill-intentioned persons and/or from indirect attacks, such as viruses.

This architecture provides for segregation of the Application Service from the Data Management Service. This segmentation makes it possible not only to physically isolate the two machines, but also to increase service redundancy.

When a hardware or software failure occurs, in view of the selectivity of provided services, the architecture will definitely be more easily and quickly restored. This also enables faster failure analysis and recovery.

Splitting services makes it possible to isolate and limit connections between Web services and DataBase services as much as possible, thus reducing exposure to the risk of programmatic and non-programmatic attacks.

A further security level is the possibility of isolating the dedicated servers for the two different services – which will be analysed below – in two separate subnets, which will be connected exclusively through routers, and where traffic can be regulated through a firewall.

Application Service

This Web service responds to "user requests" (connections through the Web or devices) in various ways, and with various data formats and types of formatting.

The Application service finally shows the user a Web browser-based Web interface which makes it possible to interact by consulting or entering data into the system.

The Application service implements a Web server which makes it possible to implement (SSL) encryption certificates through the HTTP protocol in order to encrypt the data which are transported over a HTTP protocol. In this type of set-up, sensitive data (username, password, patient data, etc.) are protected. This protocol protects communication from wiretapping/eavesdropping by generating a different encryption key for each individual transmission; this key is used to encrypt the data being transmitted in both directions. Upon every subsequent connection, a new encryption key will be generated, thus making any previous attempts to decrypt messages useless. This method is used, for instance, by electronic commerce sites to prevent wiretapping/eavesdropping of credit card numbers or any other personal data sent to the Web server.

Data Management Service

This service makes it possible to manage multilingual and multiapplication databases; services enabling multiple connections to these databases; services manag-

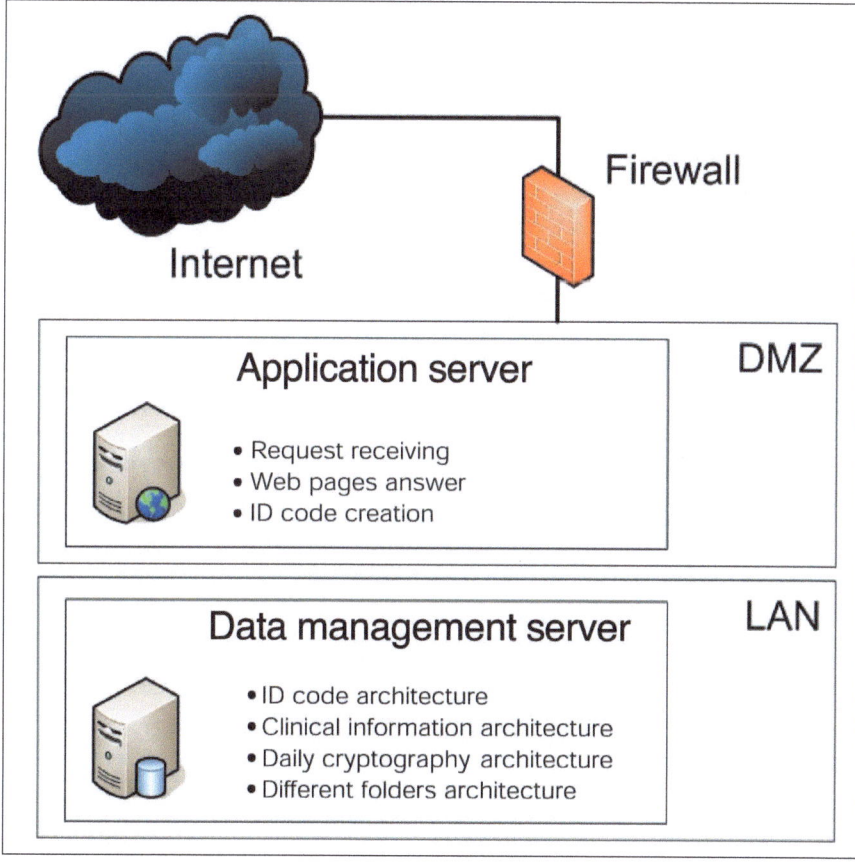

Fig. 4. Data management server

ing database filing based on backup and disaster recovery planning; and, finally, services managing database access security on a user level (Fig. 4).

Microsoft SQL Server 2000 implements all these services in a suite and a management console which is optimised for Microsoft operating systems.

In Fig. 4, attention is focussed on the division between the two levels of the service being provided.

The two levels also correspond to two Virtual LANs (VLANs) which are isolated, except for accesses, that are regulated by routers enabling connection on an IP address control and connection port level. The DMZ (or demilitarised) VLAN, where the application server is located, is the network that is exposed to the Internet, which is accessed by web clients through the HTTPS (HTTP - SSL) protocol. Given its forced exposure to the Internet, and the high risk involved in this,

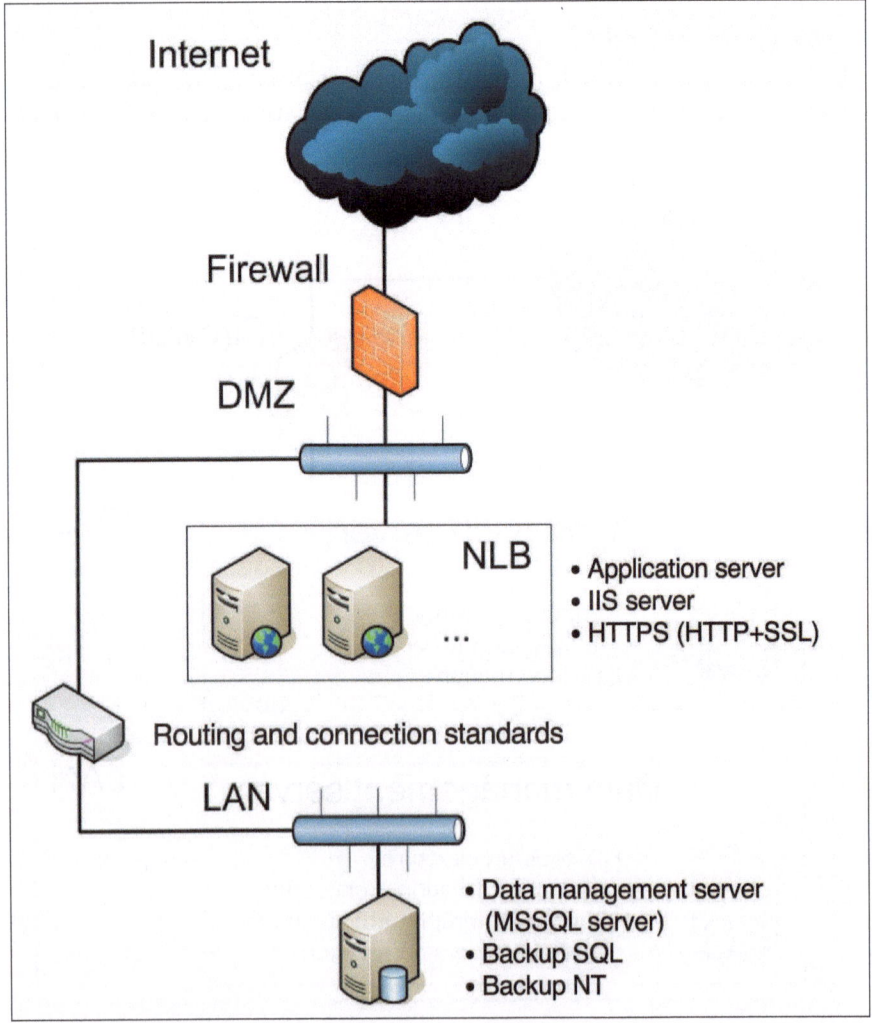

Fig. 5. Network load balancing

the DMZ VLAN is firewall-protected. Application security makes it possible to manage crucial password-related security rules. Expiry, minimum length and recurrence of passwords are managed on an application level.

Fig. 5 clarifies how the structure splits the application components described in the Application Security section.

Protection

The data concerning the network infrastructure and the servers on which the dedicated Web portal's services rely are managed through an Application server with an entry firewall to protect access to Web servers from the Internet – a network which is exposed to all kinds of attacks, whether premeditated or unpremeditated.

The Web servers located in the demilitarised area are configured under Network Load Balancing (NLB) (Fig. 5). NLB ensures both service redundancy and load balancing. In this configuration, servers can also be updated without causing any malfunction.

Thanks to the installation and configuration of Microsoft Internet Information Services, NLB Web servers ensure provision of an efficient and integrated Web service with SSL encryption security.

There is a Data Management Service where data are stored, and which has more than one database; these are associated with planned filing in order to avoid unacceptable downtimes in case of a disaster, and therefore when a situation needs to be recovered from scratch.

The data server is isolated from external connections because it is installed in a subnet, or VLAN, which is separate from the Application server's, and not directly exposed to the Internet.

Correct reception of data is ensured by an extensively proven format (XML); moreover, software securities are implemented to ensure consistency between the data which were transmitted and received by the dedicated Web portal (comparison between stored data and the data received by the server; output data will not be released until this comparison has determined that they are perfectly identical).

Data transmission from the centre (server) to the peripheral device (client) is bidirectional, and takes place through SOAP calls (XML format) over TCP-IP.

The server then posts a Web service on the Internet that is used by all remote devices to perform synchronisation. When clients connect to the Internet through a modem, they make calls according to Web service methods, thus performing data synchronisation.

Data Synchronisation

As has already been stated, the data exchange procedure is bidirectional; for this reason, the Web service makes two methods available:
- Upload Data: device data are sent to the centre.
- Download Setting: device configuration is received by the centre.

In both cases, (XML-formatted) data are transmitted in compressed binary packets, so as to minimise synchronisation time, and therefore the duration of the call which the client must make through the modem.

Data compression is performed through the Bzip2 algorithm, which generally creates files which are 60-70% as big as the corresponding files obtained using gzip. High compression also ensures correctness of data, because if even a single byte of the contents of the compressed buffer were changed, this would make it impossible to decompress it, and would thus generate an error which would prompt it to perform data transfer again.

From the moment when data are generated and sent, to the moment when they are received and saved, they go through different protocol layers (TCP-IP, HTTP, SOAP, BZIP), which check their integrity and authenticity. For this reason, once packets have been correctly received, and information has been decompressed without any errors, you are certain that transmitted and received data are the same.

The Changing Role of Nursing in Telemetric LTOT at Home

R. Bisato, C. Turati

Ever-increasing scientific knowledge and awareness of the diagnostic and therapeutic potential of medicine has led to rising expectations in terms of health and quality of life. This has, in turn, led to significant increases in health costs. On the other hand, this situation has stimulated the development of new technologies that are both clinically and economically viable, particularly for the treatment of chronic disease. Cost control without a reduction in the quality of health care has become a priority, along with the promotion of new intervention protocols developed specifically to deal with the complexity of all these factors.

In this context, the role of nursing is fundamental. The goal of nursing has always been to act as a mediator between scientific and economic values, both supporting and augmenting them, without forgetting the dignity and importance of the patient. For the nurse, the person should always come first.

Nursing process is relevant to intervention protocol formulation, especially in chronic disease care, where the clinical approach is concerned with developing long-term programs for daily self-management. These require that the patient be knowledgeable about his/her disease, allowing him/her to understand therapeutic decisions. Patients with chronic diseases should be able to access as much information as possible, allowing them to participate more actively in their treatment and to take responsibility for their disease management.

The need to provide adequate patient and caregiver education has always been one of the most important aims of nursing. This allows the patient to cope with the disease, to adhere more easily to medication protocols, to learn how to solve common problems and to manage new situations, avoiding, if possible, further hospital admissions for the same problem.

Patients on home long-term oxygen treatment (H-LTOT) have severe chronic respiratory insufficiency, usually characterised by progressive deterioration. These patients can have difficulty carrying out even the most simple daily activities. The patients suffer from frequent exacerbations and consequently require frequent hospital admissions, all of which result in very high social and economic costs.

For more than fifteen years, our Respiratory Department has followed these patients as hospitalised outpatients, assuring that they have access to hospital assistance upon their return home. In this context, we educate, plan clinical controls, organise technical assistance and deliver medications, oxygen and health care materials. This is done with the support of a telemetric system capable of transmitting in real-time and monitoring important clinical parameters on a daily basis.

When we started the project for telemetric monitoring of patients on H-LTOT in 1990, we were convinced of the need for a precise protocol [1]. This protocol has improved with experience and with periodic revision allowing it to anticipate arising needs and to resolve problems more readily.

In Italy, oxygen was recognised as a medication by the Italian Drug Formulary only in 1982 (DM 01/07/1982 GU no. 217 09/08/1982). In the years immediately following its introduction, the problem of respiratory insufficiency was epidemiologically observed and analysed in order to recognise all the different pathological conditions which necessitate H-LTOT. This included determining prescription criteria and selecting the appropriate equipment and devices for safely delivering oxygen; studying different way of storing oxygen; evaluating connection possibilities; and the best way to schedule equipment and device checks and patient clinical controls.

The project [2], supported by a grant from the *Regione Veneto* and the National Research Council (*Consiglio Nazionale delle Ricerche, CNR*) – see chapter 6 – was based on the demonstration that integrating telemedicine into this mode of treatment would reduce acute hospitalisations, thus being economically more viable for the community and more easily accepted by patients and caregivers.

From the nursing point of view, the first approach was essentially limited to evaluation of the tolerance to oxygen therapy as prescribed by the specialist and carried out by the patient, checking the effective administration time and the presence of safety and surveillance criteria. It was immediately clear that the main obstacle to successful treatment would be patient compliance. Data collected on oxygen consumption and the patient's PaO_2 and $PaCO_2$ parameters showed that improvement in a patient's condition was linked to his/her adherence to oxygen therapy: at that time 40-50% of the patients were found to substantially modify oxygen therapy schedules based mainly on their own observations, often leading to them reducing their oxygen consumption [3].

Compliance is the term frequently used within the health care system to describe the level of patient acceptance of therapeutic regimens. In the most commonly used approaches, the patient has a passive role, modifying his/her behaviour upon instruction, while the health care personnel acts as the authoritarian.

In chronic disease, the importance of patient adherence to the prescribed therapeutic regimens should not be minimised or neglected. Actually, defiance of therapeutic protocols is frequently observed, to which patients (and their caregivers) do not easily admit, and in some cases, emphatically deny. As lack of compliance is correlated with lack of the patient's understanding of, and education about their disease and treatment regimens [4], we reacted by implementing patient meetings where patients were instructed in person and via video.

The need to educate both patients and their caregivers was thus immediately perceived as crucial. How to proceed, improve and respond to this need is under continual review.

It has become evident over the years that in order to attain a patient's health potential, we need to modify the way we transmit messages about his/her disease: it is necessary to give the patient the chance to play a more active role, and to subsequently adapt his/her behaviour. This happens only if the patient is not just simply instructed, but also convinced and motivated to be the prime player in the treatment and in the maintenance of his/her health. On the other hand, medics and paramedics should abandon any authoritarian temptations, which are ineffective, and should instead adopt a more compassionate role, treating the patient as a partner.

The important role of the caregiver in supporting and encouraging patients who do not comply with treatment should not be underestimated. Any education programs directed to patients with chronic diseases should not overlook the caregiver, who is normally a close relative of the patient and can offer irreplaceable assistance in managing the disease.

Taken that patient and caregiver education on pathology and treatment is a priority, another important aspect is adherence to health prescriptions. Adherence should be checked periodically, taking into account any guilt the patient may feel about the lack of adherence to protocols and giving them the chance to explain the reasons why they may not be properly following their treatment.

The nursing role is fundamental because nurses have the correct background to understand patient needs and problems, and thus behaviour towards their disease. In addition, patients and caregivers consider the nurse as someone who can be consulted without shame, embarrassment, or fear, which allows the patient to express their opinions and clinical conditions more freely.

With the experience gained in these years, we understand that the most relevant nursing messages to give the patient regard the reasons behind low adhesion to therapeutic plans:

- *Modes of administration of inhaled medication*

Inhaled medications are difficult to use (particularly via metered dose-inhalers) and if taken incorrectly they are less effective and often harmful. Moreover, lack of education about the medication often results in lack of confidence with the medication itself; thus patients might disregard this treatment in favour of other therapeutic options.

Patients usually recognise their medication by the shape and colour of the canister rather than by the therapeutic effect of the drug; if patients use the wrong medication they might suffer from the effects of an overdose or conversely, might decide to stop the medication because they do not perceive its clinical effect.

- *Managing oxygen therapy*

Oxygen is a medication: it should be administered strictly according to the prescription (concerning dose and duration). Changes to prescribed treatment and discontinuation of treatment should be avoided.

- *Life-style*

Patients very often do not follow instructions to stop smoking, to follow an adequate diet, to limit certain activities, to pay attention to clinical signs and symptoms, all of which can result in negative consequences.

- *Nutritional aspects*

Patients with chronic obstructive pulmonary disease have been described as 'blue bloaters' and 'pink puffers'. These two extremes are very frequently met in patients on H-LTOT and our role is to reinforce motivation to follow suggested diets. Any rapid change in body weight should also be carefully monitored as it could signal a deterioration in the patient's condition.

The current intervention protocol indicates that when a patient has severe hypoxaemia and a stable clinical condition, generally after hospital admission, H-LTOT can be prescribed. The patient is then included on a list to allow them to start the home hospitalisation program.

Usually, if a patient is to access H-LTOT in the future, he/she is first contacted by the nurse while still an inpatient. After this, the patient starts an observation period [5], during which haemoglobin saturation range and pulse frequency are analysed to identify and clarify which values are normal for the patient for his/her clinical condition. Thereafter, if the patient is to be included in the H-LTOT program he/she is contacted by the telemetric and oxygen delivery services.

Patients and caregivers are instructed on the use and maintenance of the different devices and their components. During this initial stage, the importance of patient adherence to the therapeutic regimen is emphasised.

Before definitively accessing the home hospitalisation program, we try to judge the ability of the patient to:
• enter and continue a treatment program
• respect control visit appointments
• correctly administer prescribed medication
• appropriately modify his/her life-style
• accurately manage the therapeutic plan at home
• avoid behaviours that put health at risk.

Some aspects have shown to be of strategic importance for a successful education program and to obtain better adherence, these include:
• simple therapeutic schemes
• a good relationship between the physician–nurse–patient
• continuous patient and caregiver education
• good comprehension of the therapeutic treatment and of the long-term program.

Once the initial period is over, our service officially starts home hospitalisation and a clinical folder and a computerised nursing folder are created. Finally, the telemetric software is updated and timings and limits for parameter measurements are planned [6]. The system offers the possibility to design questionnaires that can be sent to the patient telemetrically, giving us the chance to understand problems that might occur and which could lead to deterioration in patient quality of life.

A schedule is then planned for the next outpatient controls. At the time of the control, the nurse verifies if the patient has correctly taken the medication according to the therapeutic plan and if the devices have been correctly maintained. The nurse then gives medication to the patient to last until the next planned clinical control. The nurse must determine if the patient has encountered new problems and, if necessary, he/she acts as a liaison between the patient and the specialist.

Although medicine is driven by productivity, nurses should always take the time to listen.

When discussing chronic diseases, and in particular incurable diseases, treatment should be considered as a means of improving the disease condition, rather than as a cure. This fact needs to be accepted and understood by all those involved in the health plan.

Treatment should be addressed towards prevention of symptoms and exacerbations, thus limiting the effects of the disease on the overall health state of the patient. Moreover, the disease itself is often associated with other relevant pathological conditions such as cardiovascular disease, hypertension etc.; in these cases it is particularly important to treat the patient holistically [7].

It is important to let the patient conduct his/her life as normally as possible, even in the most difficult cases, where patients have problems attempting even the most simple daily activities, such as washing and dressing. It is thus necessary to widen clinical evaluation from the traditional biomedical parameters in order to consider functional, physical, mental and social capacities, especially as they are perceived by the patient.

Disease symptoms include not only bronchoconstriction, dyspnoea, cough and phlegm, but also sleep disturbance, fatigue, as well as altered psychological status. All these have physical and emotional effects and can have a strong impact on the perception of health status.

The nurse should be able to act as a technical interface, collecting all possible information and then elaborating on it and transmitting the most relevant messages to the patient, the caregivers and the staff of specialists who are in charge of the patient.

Attaining the planned assistance goals, which we consider necessary for a better quality of life, depends on two variables [8]: first, the capacity to begin, maintain and reinforce the relationship between the health care personnel and the patient and second, the effectiveness of the educational messages transmitted within this relationship.

Actually, even though it is the specialist physician who should primarily act as the educator, it is the nurse who is responsible for widening, reinforcing, and implementing this education.

At present, our service has 289 patients enrolled in H-LTOT, 166 of whom are followed within the home hospitalisation program. Patients involved in this program feel that they are fundamental partners in their health care process and for this reason they participate more actively in their therapeutic plans. They feel confident that they have the possibility to signal any change in their health status immediately and can transmit important parameters telemetrically.

Telemetry is competently put into practice and appreciated by the patients, despite initial fears of difficulties in patients with little technological expertise. On the contrary, patients often request telemetry as they perceive it as a valid way for them to understand the severity and urgency of any exacerbations more quickly.

Over the years, this approach has shown to be a useful support instrument for managing a very debilitating disease. The effectiveness of the project is demonstrated by the number of satisfied patients, a reduction in the number of hospital admissions and, when these cannot be avoided, reduction in the length of hospital stays [9]. This success, in turn, acts as a constant stimulus for us to review our strategies in order to make the program more effective and productive.

References

1. Dal Negro RW, Pomari C, Micheletto C (1995) Ossigenoterapia domiciliare a lungo termine (OTLT) sotto controllo telematico: aspetti farmacoeconomici. Farmacoeconomia 2(4):43-46
2. Dal Negro RW, Turco P, Pomari C (1991) Progetto di telemetria per l'home care respiratorio. Risultati preliminari. Rass Pat App Resp 6(1):111
3. Earnest MA (2002) Explaining adherence to supplemental oxygen therapy: the patient's perspective. J Gen Intern Med 17(10):749-755
4. Gibbons D, Conneelly J, Smith J (2002) An audit of provision of long-term oxygen therapy for COPD patients. Prof Nurse 18(2):107-110
5. Andersson I, Johansson K, Larsson S, Pehrsson K (2002) Long-term oxygen therapy and quality of life in elderly patients hospitalised due to severe exacerbation of COPD. A 1-year follow-up study. Respir Med 96(11):944-949
6. Dal Negro RW, Turco P, Pomari C (1992) A telemetric system for respiratory home care. 2nd International Congress on Advances in Pulmonary Rehabilitation and Management of Chronic Respiratory Failure. Proceedings, p 156
7. Micheletto C, Pomari C, Dal Negro RW (1995) Analisi delle cause di mortalità in un quadriennio di LTOT. GIMT Proc, p 101
8. Eaton T, Lewis C, Young P, Kennedy Y, Garrett JE, Kolbe J (2004) Long-term oxygen therapy improves health-related quality of life. Respir Med 98(4):285-293
9. Dal Negro RW (2000) Long term oxygen tele-home monitoring, the Italian perspective. Chest 2000 Companion Book, pp 247-249

Home LTOT: Patient–Caregiver Compliance and Adhesion

P. Pescatori, R. Cadinu

Qualitative improvement of health services is essential in order to offer a level of assistance that can respond to the evolving needs of patients. The current National Health Service (NHS) law (DL 502/1992 and 517/2003) states that the qualitative evaluation of health services is fundamental. Article 14, which concerns the rights of citizens suffering from any disease, is of particular importance as it imposes the adoption of Quality indicators concerning the customisation of assistance, the right of information, food and accommodation services, and activities directed towards disease prevention. From the point of view of this evolution, the patient, or better, the client/customer, takes on a central and crucial role around which the different health organisation responsibilities move (Fig. 1).

The assessment and monitoring of patient satisfaction requires the personal commitment of a health care professional in order to build up a Quality system as a basis for continuing Quality improvement (Fig. 2).

Around this cultural evolution we would like to highlight two aspects that are equally important and tightly-linked. The first is the search for efficacy and efficiency of the offered health service; that is, the ability to find the most appropriate

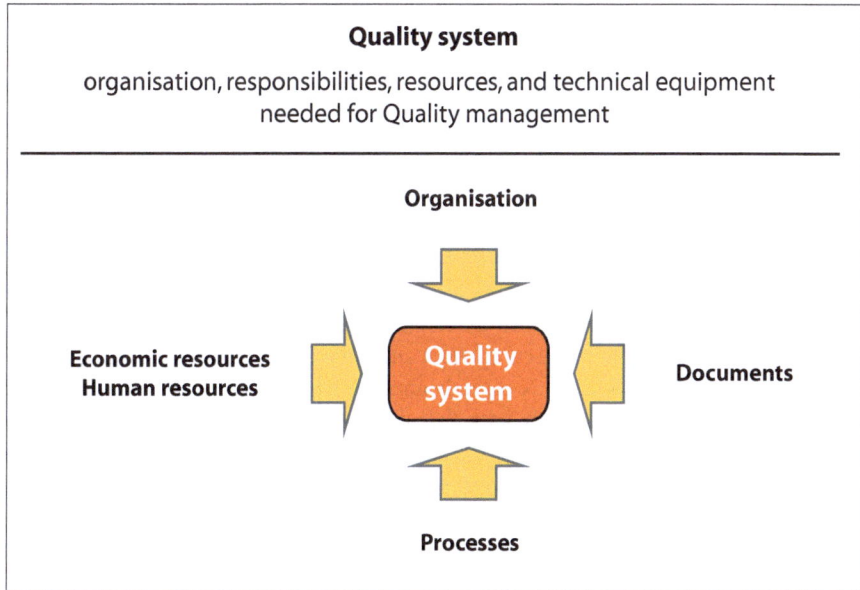

Fig. 1. Quality system architecture

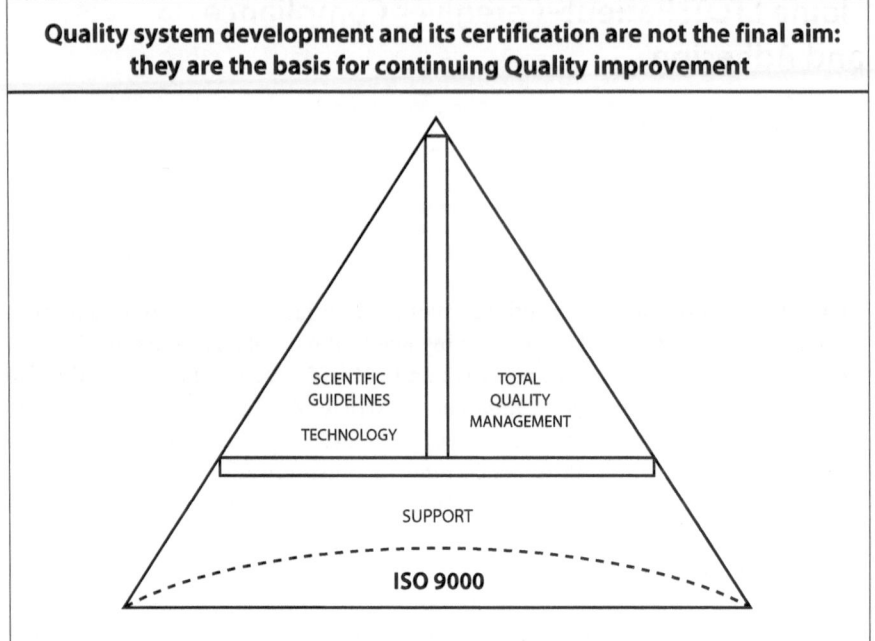

Quality system development and its certification are not the final aim: they are the basis for continuing Quality improvement

SCIENTIFIC GUIDELINES
TECHNOLOGY

TOTAL QUALITY MANAGEMENT

SUPPORT

ISO 9000

Fig. 2. Quality system is the basis for continuing Quality improvement

therapeutic strategies for each customer, and to offer them in the shortest time and using minimal resources. The second aspect that can be highlighted within this process of continuing improvement concerns quality of life. In other words, consolidating the patient's degree of independence and his/her possibility to retain social activities and relationships.

It is important to note that society members themselves have come to play a more central role in the management of their own health. However, as reported in this book, the patient needs to be accompanied and supported by health personnel in this process (Fig. 3).

In fact, the role of specialist nursing has become increasingly important; it is indispensable for the education of the patient about his/her disease, its consequences, and its impact on quality of life, in addition to managing the therapeutic plan. Within this context, particular attention should be paid to the role of the families, who are more and more involved in disease management to the point where they effectively become caregivers, and thus active protagonists within the therapeutic treatment. They care directly about the health needs of the patient and they assist the patient to comply with therapeutic protocols (Fig. 4).

The caregiver's role is central to disease management and it has even more relevance when it is linked to the treatment of chronic disease and particularly, of chronic respiratory disease. This is because treatment of chronic respiratory disease necessitates continual drug administration and life-style changes in order to obtain the necessary therapeutic goals. In these cases, the caregiver's role is often central not only for the technical reasons that we will discuss later, but also for pro-

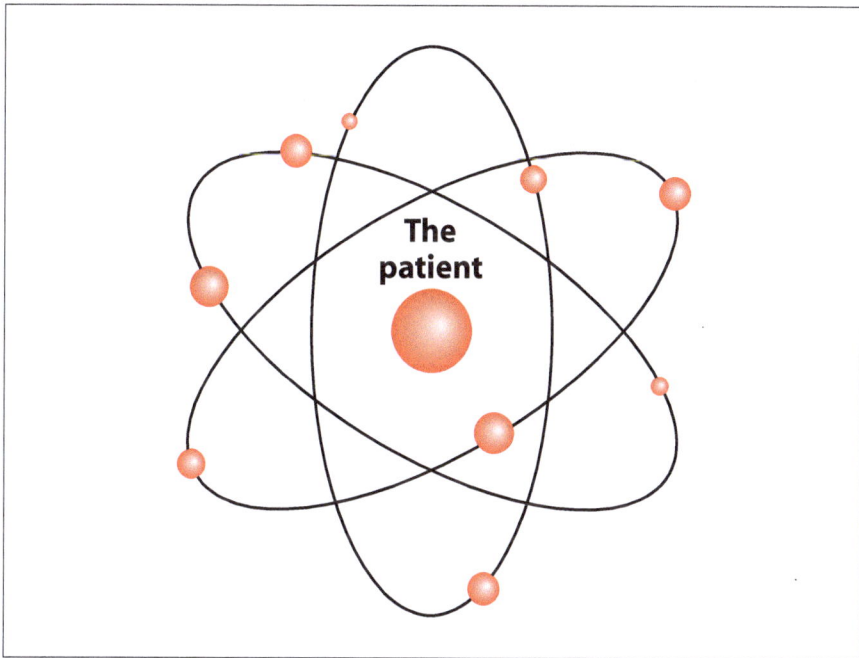

Fig. 3. The patient is in the center of nursing activities

viding the constant psychological support that these patients need (Fig. 5).

There is often a gap between patient expectation and achievement of therapeutic goals. These goals do not aim to cure the patient, but rather to improve general health status and to prevent acute events. Within this context, the psychologi-

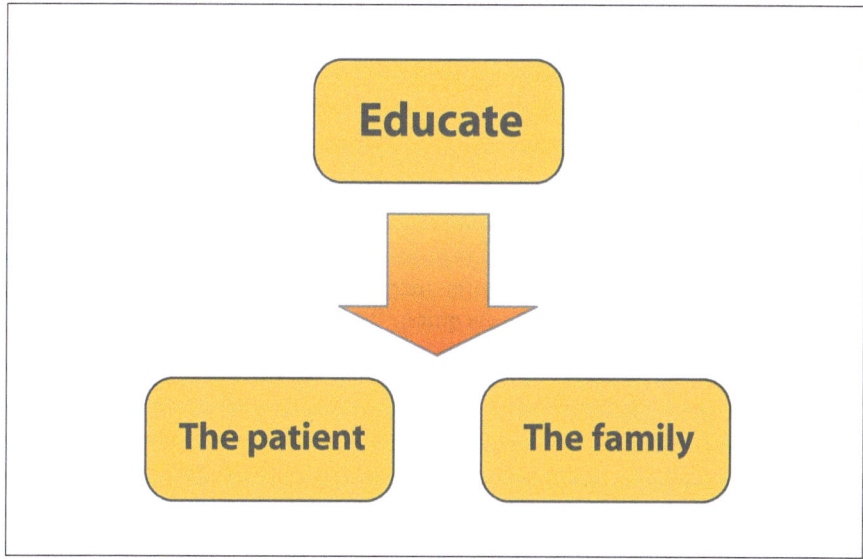

Fig. 4. Continuous education of the patient and caregiver improves compliance

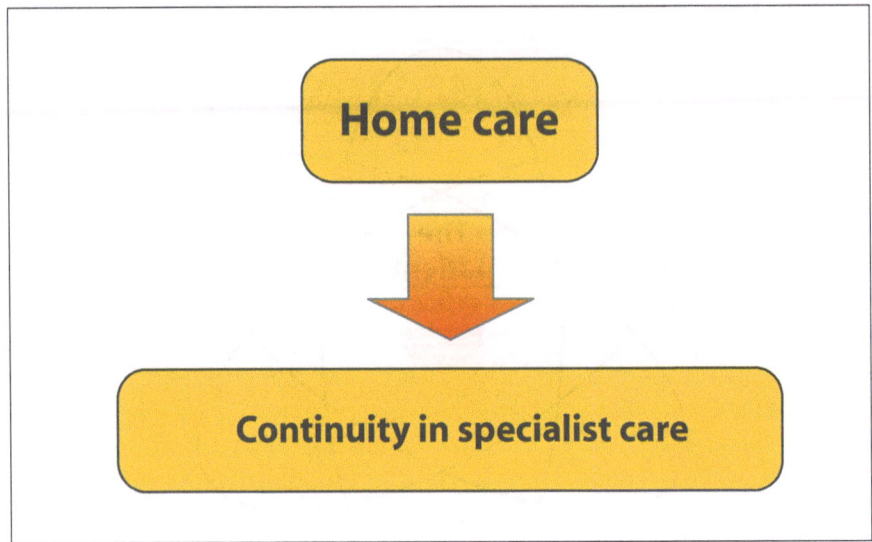

Fig. 5. Assistance moves towards a home-based model

cal status of the patient might have a detrimental effect on their adhesion to therapeutic treatments in the long-term. Therefore, the caregiver acts as an irreplaceable positive stimulus and psychological support for the patient.

Health personnel can thus not ignore compliance of the patient/caregiver couple or their willingness to collaborate and adhere to therapeutic plans. This necessitates the adoption of professional strategies to improve compliance, in particular:

- simple therapeutic schemes
- a good physician—nurse—patient relationship
- continuous education of the patient and caregiver
- verification of treatment comprehension in the long-term.

A crucial point to consider is the process of educating the patient and caregiver, which requires specific pedagogic knowledge. It is necessary to propose educational plans that are appropriate to the patient's disease and to consider progressive transfer of therapeutic competency from the health professionals to the patient and/or his/her caregiver, thus promoting autonomy and active collaboration.

Through our Specialist Centre, which provides education to patients affected by respiratory insufficiency undergoing long-term oxygen treatment (LTOT), we have established that these patients acquire:

- a knowledge of their disease and related medications
- the capability to carry out procedures useful to treatment
- the ability to be helped by caregivers that follow a parallel training.

The utility and necessity of continuous and appropriate education has become even more relevant, considering that assistance is moving more and more towards a home-based model. This is a model that our Specialist Centre supports as a strategic choice and has been practising for many years (Fig. 6).

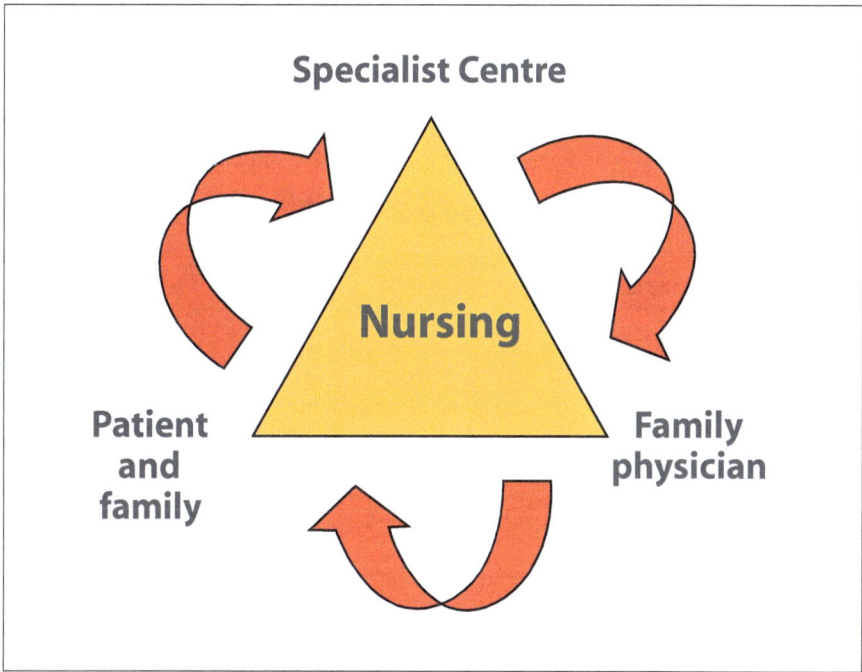

Fig. 6. Nursing role in patient's assistance

Many of our patients, particularly those on LTOT, follow a 'hospitalised home' regime. In these cases, it is obvious that the education of the patient and caregiver about therapy is of prime importance. At the start of the therapy, we establish a module for data collection in the patient's home; this module can, via normal telephone lines, send parameters such as oxymetry values, oxygen consumption and heart frequency to our Specialist Centre, thus giving us the possibility to maintain a constant telemetric evaluation of the patient's status, especially important in more complex cases. This technology not only gives the patient the ability to send an SOS message to the hospital, but its adoption has offered us the chance to monitor patients more carefully and has given us the opportunity to acquire important data on disease progression. On the other hand, use of this technology requires specific training in the correct use of software, hardware and other devices.

This treatment model necessitates a training program that includes instructions on:
- device and accessory use given in the patient's home
- respiratory medication administration (in particular, correct utilisation of metered-dose inhalers and dry powder inhalers)
- adhesion to prescribed therapies
- stroller utilisation
- possible life-style changes.

In the first phase, it is necessary to monitor compliance of the patient/caregiver couple strictly, and to initiate a close collaboration with the health team: future

Table 1. LTOT questionnaire for patient/caregivers

Who is the caregiver?	53.5% partner
	23.3% other
	19.7% son/daughter
	3.5% brother/sister
Caregiver's average age	54.9±12.8 SD
Individuals within the family	2.4±0.9 SD

Table 2. For how many hours do you use oxygen during the day?

	Patient response	Caregiver response
Morning	2.8±2.3 SD	3.1±2.3 SD
Afternoon	4.6±2.4 SD	4.9±2.3 SD
Night	7.9±0.2 SD	7.3±2.1 SD

results will depend on the quality of this cooperation. Following the initial period, LTOT patients with difficult and complex clinical conditions are admitted to 'domiciliary hospitalisation' and all their medical controls are planned strictly as in the case of regular hospitalisation.

To evaluate the relationship between our Specialist Hospital Unit and the patient/caregiver couple more effectively, we devised a questionnaire for patients and their caregivers. From this survey, we determined that daily management of patients on LTOT is essentially carried out by close relatives of the patient rather than employed personnel (Table 1). Within the family, the most involved person is usually the patient's partner (53.5% of the cases). This person is obviously not a health care professional and the quality of the care that they give depends mostly on their age and health.

Within our program for managing patients on LTOT, specialist nursing activity in the last three years has been specifically aimed at obtaining the best possible adherence to oxygen therapy prescription regarding both schedule and flow. As reported in Table 2, it became evident that oxygen therapy is mostly carried out during the afternoon and at night, information independently confirmed by the patient and caregiver. Moreover, thanks to nursing care, there has been an increase in the number of patients who correctly respond to respiratory distress by increasing the period over which they take oxygen. However, despite our repeated recommendations, some patients still respond by increasing oxygen flow (Table 3).

Another crucial point of specialist nursing for LTOT concerns oxygen stroller acceptance and utilisation. Correct use of the stroller has the potential to increase patient autonomy. In the last three years, there has been an increase in the use of this type of device, both inside (Table 4) and outside (Table 5) the home. This suggests that patients have become more comfortable with using a device that displays their disability, signalling that the disability itself is becoming better accept-

Table 3. What do you do when you have increased respiratory distress?

	Patient response	Caregiver response
Increase O_2 hours	50.0%	57.1%
Increase O_2 flow	19.2%	23.8%
Increase MDI or DPI use	15.3%	19.1%
Other	15.5%	—

MDI, metered-dose inhalers; DPI, dry powder inhalers

Table 4. Do you use the stroller at home?

	Patient response		Caregiver response	
	2002	2004	2002	2004
Always	25.0%	50.0%	21.4%	53.8%
Sometimes	28.5%	26.8%	2.4%	23.0%
Never	46.4%	23.0%	53.5%	23.0%

Table 5. Do you use the stroller when you go outside?

	Patient response		Caregiver response	
	2002	2004	2002	2004
Always	10.7%	46.2%	28.5%	46.2%
Sometimes	25.0%	30.8%	39.2%	23.0%
Never	60.7%	23.0%	28.5%	30.8%

Table 6. If you use the stroller, who charges it?

	Patient response		Caregiver response	
	2002	2004	2002	2004
A relative	61.5%	33.0%	48.0%	41.7%
The patient	34.0%	25.0%	52.0%	33.0%
Others	—	41.7%	—	24.0%

ed by society. In fact, when we ask patients why they do not use the stroller, the percentage responding "I do not feel comfortable" has dropped from 50% to 15.4% in patients, and from 70% to 30.8% in caregivers, over a period of three years. Stroller management is mainly the responsibility of the caregiver and only in a minority of cases does the patient seems to have the ability to manage it himself/herself (Table 6). This confirms that caregiver education is still very important in order to attain good home management of LTOT patients.

Finally, the importance of the customer/caregiver couple within the health plan must be addressed in order to obtain optimal patient adhesion to therapeutic protocols that are becoming increasingly detailed and complex. In our experience, the participation of the caregiver has led to an improvement in the management of the disease and thus in the quality of life of the patient, even if such participation requires increased resources and is more time-consuming.

Suggested Reading

1. Dal Negro R, Farina M (a cura di) (2005) L'approccio e la gestione per processi in pneumologia. Aspetti applicativi secondo il modello ISO 9001:2000. Springer-Verlag, Milano
2. Dal Negro R, Farina M (2003) L'applicazione pratica del modello ISO 9001:2000 in ambito pneumologico. Centro Scientifico Editore, Torino
3. Pescatori P (2002) OTLT domiciliare: compliance e adesione del binomio paziente-care giver. Atti del congresso "Asma bronchiale: nuovi obiettivi nuovi rimedi", Verona
4. Petty TL, Casaburi R (2000) Recommendations of the fifth Oxygen Consensus Conference. Writing and Organizing Committees. Respir Care 45(8):957-961

Complications in LTOT patients

C. Micheletto, R. W. Dal Negro

Two landmark studies, the Nocturnal Oxygen Therapy Trial (NOTT) [1] and the British Medical Research Council (MRC) trial [2] have clearly shown that long-term oxygen therapy (LTOT) improves survival in patients with severe chronic obstructive pulmonary disease (COPD) associated with resting hypoxaemia. In both studies, it has been shown that the more continuous the therapy, the better the survival rate. The precise mechanism by which continuous LTOT improves survival is not well understood, however it could be explained by effects on several haemodynamic variables.

Although the cause of death in patients with hypoxic cor pulmonale is uncertain, the factors predicting survival in patients on LTOT have been investigated. In general, variables reflecting severity of COPD, such as reduction of PaO_2 or increased $PaCO_2$ [3], lower FEV1 [4] and elevated mean pulmonary artery pressure [4] correlate inversely with survival. The most important evidence supporting the use of chronic oxygen has been derived from studies investigating its effect on survival [5]. In 1970, Neff and Petty [6] found a 30-40% decrease in mortality in their severely hypoxic patients on continuous oxygen compared with those in the literature. LTOT is one of the few interventions in patients with COPD that improves survival when used for more than 15 hours per day [1]. LTOT has also been shown to have a number of important physiological benefits, although it has little effect on other factors, including health-related quality of life or reduction in disease exacerbations. Many COPD patients exhibit marked abnormalities in overnight ventilation, with a consequent derangement of blood gases and ventilatory muscle dysfunction, which may contribute to the progressive deterioration seen in this group.

Pulmonary Hypertension as a Complication of COPD Patients during LTOT

Pulmonary hypertension (PH) is a common complication of advanced COPD. It develops as a result of chronic alveolar hypoxia leading to the remodelling of the pulmonary arterial wall [7, 8] and may be latent and easily unmasked by exercise. In the past, PH was found to be an important prognostic factor for COPD [9, 10]. Most patients with COPD have mild or moderate PH at rest. Unfortunately, the severely inflated lung tissue makes the echocardiographic evaluation of PH technically very difficult. The first trial with prolonged oxygen treatment in patients with severe COPD was conducted to assess its effects on pulmonary arterial pressure (PAP) [11, 12]. The results were very encouraging. A significant reduction in PH was observed after several weeks of continuous or 15 to 17 hours per day of oxygen treatment [13-15]. Oxygen supplementation may act on a number of different levels to reduce exercise-induced PH; it is likely that oxygen decreases dyspnoea, perhaps by decreasing the respiratory rate during exercise allowing for a better emptying of the lung and less auto-positive end expiratory pressure, and it may decrease the sympathetic tone.

Investigations on sustained use of LTOT also showed positive results. Stark et al. [16] observed a fall in mean PAP by 12 mmHg after eight months of LTOT given for 15 hours per day in COPD patients. Cooper et al. [17] found a decrease in PAP by 2.2 mmHg after one year of LTOT for 15 hours per day in 40 COPD patients. All these studies, however, were not controlled and used relatively small numbers of patients.

Two controlled studies, oxygen treatment group versus no oxygen group (MRC) [2], or continuous oxygen versus nocturnal oxygen (NOTT) [1], were compared. In the first study, patients breathing with oxygen for 15 hours per day showed the stabilisation of PAP during almost two years of treatment. In patients from the control group (no oxygen), PAP increased by 2.8 mmHg per year.

In the NOTT trial, patients treated with continuous oxygen (18 hours per day) demonstrated a fall in PAP by 3 mmHg, whereas no change in PAP was observed in patients receiving oxygen for 12 hours. The second measurements were performed after six months of oxygen treatment.

A long prospective study describing the effects of breathing supplemental oxygen on pulmonary haemodynamics in patients with severe COPD, complicated by hypoxic PH, has clearly shown that LTOT administered for approximately 14 hours per day induces a small reduction of PH during the first two years of LTOT [18]. Thereafter, PH returned to the initial level and showed stabilisation over six years. The long-term stabilisation of PH occurred despite progression of the airflow limitation and of hypoxaemia. The reason for limited effects of oxygen on pulmonary vasculature may be an insufficient number of oxygen-breathing hours. The MRC and NOTT studies showed better effects on pulmonary haemodynamics for 18 versus 15 hours of oxygen [1, 2].

Complete normalisation of PAP rarely occurred, but the changes in PAP were related to differences in pulmonary vascular resistance. The importance of PH as a predictor of death suggests that LTOT could be prescribed earlier for COPD patients with cor pulmonale, as oxygen has been shown to be the only effective therapy for improving the survival probability of the patients.

Histopathologic studies of the pulmonary arteries of patients who died after being treated with domiciliary oxygen have shown persistent structural changes. These were especially evident in the intima of small pulmonary arteries and arterioles [19, 20]. There is no evidence so far that LTOT is able to eliminate the noncellular irreversible intimal fibroelastosis [21].

Many patients' conditions continue to worsen despite long-term oxygen treatment. Early identification of those patients who are unlikely to benefit from oxygen would avoid cost and inconvenience. Patients who have an acute haemodynamic response to oxygen may have structural differences in their pulmonary vasculature compared with those who do not improve. However, an autopsy study examining the pulmonary arteries of patients who died during the NOTT study found no difference in the vascular structure of those who responded to oxygen and those who did not.

Clotting and Thrombosis in COPD during LTOT

The pulmonary arteries in COPD patients are characterised by endothelial cell dysfunction. Cytokines like interleukin (IL)-1 and IL-6 have been shown to be increased in the plasma of patients with COPD. These, and also oxidative stress and C-reactive protein, may affect endothelial cell function and render the endothelium a more thrombogenic surface. In fact, a hypercoagulable state has been described in patients with severe COPD [22]. There appears to be an increased frequency of deep venous thrombosis and pulmonary embolism in acute exacerbation of COPD [22], and thrombotic lesions were detected histopathologically in lung tissue from patients with severe emphysema undergoing lung-volume reduction surgery [23]. Apparently, the frequency of venous thrombosis is increased during exacerbations of COPD. Clearly the clotting and embolism aspects of COPD, especially during an exacerbation, require further investigations. The inflammatory aspects of the so-called COPD exacerbations may trigger a hypercoagulable state and increase the risk of thrombosis. Some *post mortem* studies indicate that a considerable number of patients dying with COPD have pulmonary embolic events. Should indeed a hypercoagulable state, or pulmonary embolism, or *in situ* thrombosis be frequent events in patients with severe COPD, then anti-coagulants could be a possible therapy.

Chronic Respiratory Failure

Long-term domiciliary oxygen prolongs life in patients with COPD, despite inexorable progression of airflow limitation and of hypoxaemia. One of the beneficial effects of oxygen is an elimination of alveolar hypoxia. This prevents progression of PH and development of clinical signs of cor pulmonale. In the 1950s, a great number of COPD patients were dying from right heart failure [24]. It seems that the advent of LTOT changed this picture. A more recent multicenter study on causes and circumstances of death in COPD patients undergoing LTOT showed that only 13% died from right heart failure [25]. Of the 215 patients evaluated, the major causes of death were: acute or chronic respiratory failure (38%), heart failure (13%), pulmonary infection (11%), pulmonary embolism (10%), cardiac arrhythmia (8%) and lung cancer (7%). A lower arterial carbon dioxide tension, less oxygen usage and increased incidence of arrhythmias were seen in those patients who died suddenly. Drug therapy was not related to unexpected death. The majority of patients with COPD on LTOT died from chronic or acute chronic respiratory failure. Prevention and treatment of respiratory failure is likely to have the greatest impact in reducing mortality.

Patients with COPD are frequently admitted to hospital with episodes of acute exacerbations of their disease, characterised by hypoxaemia and respiratory acidosis, the latter resulting to a large part from a rapid shallow pattern of breathing, despite strong respiratory efforts by the patients. Non-invasive ventilation has the potential of partially reversing these abnormalities. Data obtained during face or nose mask pressure-support ventilation both in stable and in acutely ill COPD patients showed that this technique was able to reduce diaphragmatic activity, to improve gas exchange and tended to normalise the breathing pattern [26]. A combination of oxygen therapy plus nasal intermittent positive pressure ventilation at home improved blood gases in spontaneous ventilation as well as the quality of life of patients with COPD [27].

Acute Exacerbations

The natural history of COPD is one of a progressive decline in ventilatory function, exercise capacity, and health status that is punctuated with varying frequency by exacerbations of symptoms. Exacerbations have major effects on health status and are associated with considerable morbidity and mortality [28], and often lead to hospital admission, representing a major component of the socio-economic burden related to COPD [29]. The aetiology of acute exacerbations of COPD is complex, including mucous plugging and regional atelectasis, inhalation of environmental irritants, discontinuation of medications, deviation from diet, viral infection, atypical bacteria, and common bacterial infection [30]. In our experience, in more than 40% of COPD exacerbations no infectious agent was recognised; bacterial pathogens were isolated only in 1/3 of subjects. In these cases, Gram-negative bacteria are the most common agents; in about 1/4 of cases, the infection was related only to viruses, RSV being the most common, also in adults [31] (Figs. 1, 2).

Even though the precise role of bacterial infection in the course and the pathogenesis of COPD has been a source of controversy for decades, bacteria have a crucial role in the pathogenesis of COPD exacerbations. Bacteria may be isolated during periods of quiescence, but quantitative cultures have demonstrated an increase of some pathogens during acute exacerbations [32]. Moreover, bacteria can cause direct epithelial damage, and bacterial endotoxin has been shown to increase epithelial expression of some pro-inflammatory cytokines *in vitro*, providing a

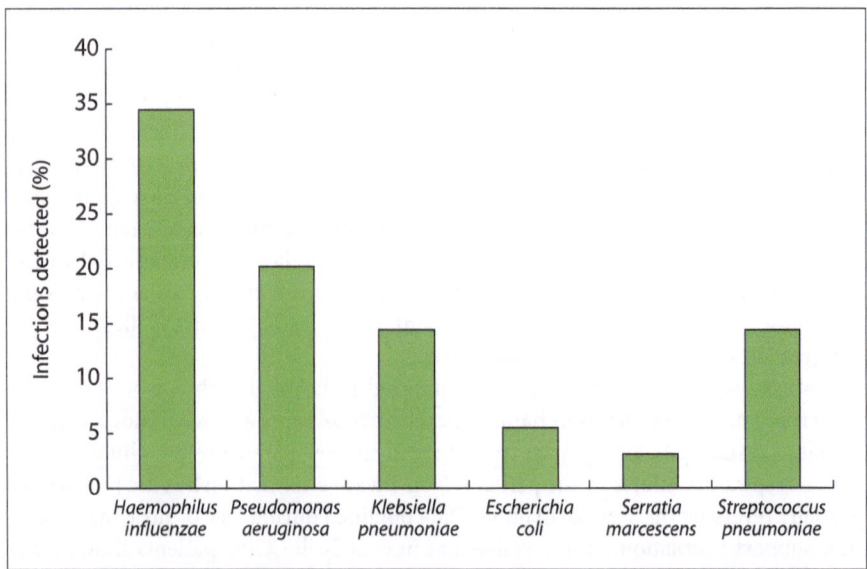

Fig. 1. Bacteria isolated from patients with COPD exacerbation

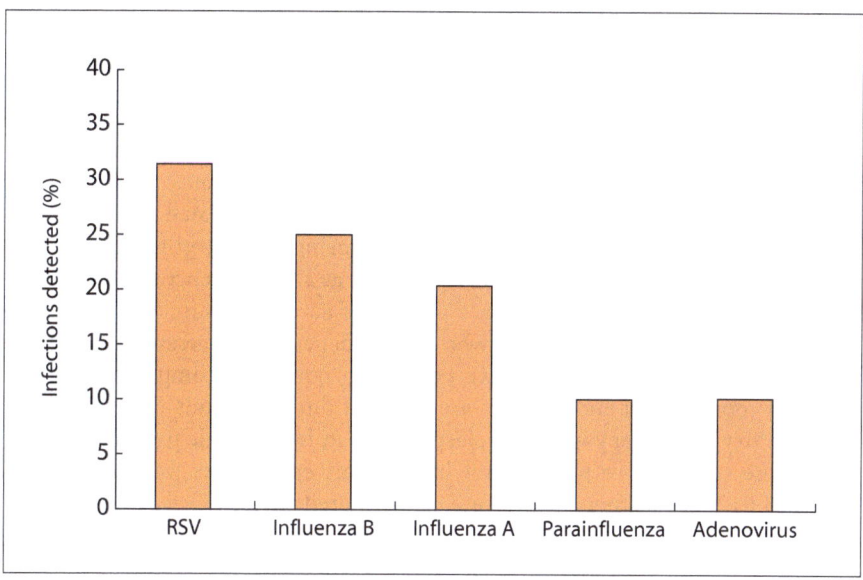

Fig. 2. Viruses isolated from patients with COPD exacerbations

potential mechanism to upregulate inflammation. Viral infections are also important triggers for COPD exacerbations, which are frequently triggered by upper respiratory tract infections. When exacerbated, COPD subjects express different patterns of pro-inflammatory mediators in bronchial secretions, which appear to be modulated according to the etiological cause of the exacerbations [33]. In particular, TNFα concentration *per se* enables recognition of COPD exacerbations due to *Pseudomonas aeruginosa*, while levels of IL-8 and IL1β prove helpful in discriminating exacerbations due to common bacteria from those due to viral agents and to non-infectious causes. The use of a decisional rule based on cytokine measurements might be regarded as a helpful predictive tool, supporting rapid clinical decisions made at the bedside regarding the best therapeutic strategy for COPD exacerbations, in particular in severe COPD patients [33].

Airway bacterial colonisation has been shown to be related to the degree of airflow obstruction and whether the patient is a smoker [34].

The type of bacterial species was related to the degree of inflammation, with *Pseudomonas aeruginosa* colonisation showing greater neutrophilic inflammation [35].

Pneumonia is a severe cause of acute respiratory failure in LTOT patients with severe COPD [36] and a frequent reason for hospitalisation. There is a better survival rate of LTOT patients with pneumonia for those who have a precise surveillance of oxygen therapy by telemedicine and a rational antibiotics protocol [36].

Sleep Disorders

The mechanisms of hypoxaemia during sleep in COPD include hyperventilation, a reduction in functional residual capacity, and alterations in ventilation-perfusion matching. The major cause of hypoxaemia during REM sleep is hypoventilation, which appears related to rapid shallow breathing and long episodes of hypopnoeas [37]. In addition, both the hypoxic and hypercapnic ventilatory responses are diminished [38]. Hypercapnia may be worsened overnight with the addition of supplemental oxygen therapy.

An acute elevation of CO_2 tension in arterial blood during the night may contribute to arousal and thus impaired sleep quality. The cause of REM sleep hypoventilation has not been fully determined, but appears related to altered brain stem function during phasic neuronal activity. During REM sleep, the ribcage contribution to ventilation decreases by 18-34% [38] as a consequence of hypotonia of the intercostal muscles and decreased activity of accessory muscles. This may be important in patients with COPD who greatly depend on accessory muscles for breathing. Patients with COPD have poor sleep quality as compared with age-matched controls [39] and arousals are frequent during periods of desaturation. Whether oxygen therapy improves sleep quality in hypoxaemic patients is debatable; some studies have found fewer hypoxaemic episodes as well as increased total and REM sleep when patients are administered oxygen.

Neuropsychologic Effects of Hypoxia

Even mild hypoxia can impair judgement, learning and short-term memory in normal subjects. To investigate the effects of chronic hypoxaemia, research has focussed on the neurobehavioral effects of hypoxaemia in patients with COPD. Early work by Krop and colleagues [40] demonstrated poorer neuropsychological performance in a group of COPD patients with a PaO_2 below 55 mmHg. Two large multicenter studies in the United States and Canada examined the neuropsychologic consequences of hypoxaemia [41, 42]. The US Nocturnal Oxygen Therapy Trial studied 203 patients with a mean age of 64 years and PaO_2 of 51 torr and found that 42% of patients had moderate to severe impairment of cerebral function [41]. The Canadian IPPB Trial examined 100 patients with less hypoxaemia (mean PaO_2 of 66 torr) which resulted in more severe impairment [42]. The results of both these studies were combined, demonstrating an increase in the rate of deficits from 27% in mild hypoxaemia (PaO_2 >60) to 61% in severe hypoxaemia (PaO_2 <50).

The poor neuropsychologic performance in hypoxaemic COPD patients has been explained by weakness, fatigue and depression. However, there is increasing evidence that brain hypoxia itself is responsible for the impaired function. Some studies suggest that hypoxia can result in reduced synthesis of acetylcholine from labelled precursors [43], which is interesting, since there is growing evidence to support the role of acetylcholine in memory and learning.

Nutritional Depletion in Patients on LTOT

The association between nutritional depletion and chronic respiratory disease has been recognised for many years and has been clearly documented in COPD. The prevalence of nutritional depletion in patients with severe COPD is quite variable, according to the method of nutritional assessment and the population studied.

Malnutrition is frequent in patients with advanced disease, especially those with severe airflow obstruction, emphysema, or chronic hypoxaemia. In this setting, body weight loss and muscle wasting have an impact on physical performance and respiratory muscle function and are responsible for an increase in health care requirements independent of the degree of airflow obstruction [44]. Nutritional depletion is also an independent risk factor for mortality and hospitalisation in patients with COPD receiving LTOT [45]. In addition to the consequences of low body weight on mortality, malnutrition has been shown to be related to morbidity in acutely ill patients with COPD. COPD patients show an increased need for mechanical ventilation in acute exacerbations, increased risk of early non-elective readmission in patients previously admitted for an exacerbation and increased duration of ventilatory support [45].

Malnutrition is highly prevalent in home-assisted respiratory patients in LTOT and is related to causal disease, FEV1, smoking and disability. Fat-free mass and fat mass, expressed as a percent of the ideal body weight, is a more sensitive measure than the body mass index for detecting malnutrition and showed better correlation with ventilatory pump use and disability. Airflow obstruction and smoking habits appeared to be independent determinants of malnutrition [46].

Hazards of Home Oxygen Therapy

Oxygen toxicity, CO_2 retention and the possibility of accidents during the storage and handling of oxygen are the main hazards of home oxygen therapy. It is not known if oxygen toxicity occurs during LTOT. Petty et al. [47], in an uncontrolled autopsy study, have reported exudative and proliferative changes in the lungs consistent with oxygen toxicity in patients with LTOT. However, the widely accepted benefits of LTOT on survival and quality of life outweigh the remote risk of oxygen toxicity.

Carbon monoxide retention is uncommon during LTOT, especially when the titration of the oxygen setting leads to a PaO_2 of 60-65 mmHg. Though the precise mechanism of O_2-induced CO_2 retention is not clear, it is relatively uncommon when oxygen in the inspired air is 35-40%. It is more common and more likely to be severe in patients with acute exacerbations, particularly in those with CO_2 retention before O_2 therapy is administered [48]. Finally, O_2-induced CO_2 retention can occur only in patients who cannot increase their ventilation appropriately with increases in $PaCO_2$.

Oxygen is neither explosive nor combustible, but because it does support combustion its potential fire hazards must be recognised. Several accidents involving fires and explosions have been reported during home oxygen therapy [49]. The majority of those accidents have been caused by patients lighting cigarettes during oxygen therapy. Neither patients nor bystanders are allowed to smoke during LTOT. Oxygen cylinders or reservoirs should not be stored near heat or flame sources. Liquid oxygen should be handled with care to avoid serious freeze burns.

Finally, it is important to note that compressed oxygen cylinders should be fixed correctly to avoid accidental falls or explosive disconnection of the regulators. This is necessary in order to avoid malfunction of the devices or unnecessary interventions by the patient or the family. The safe use of oxygen in the home requires that patients and their families be knowledgeable about its hazards.

References

1. Medical Research Council Working Group (1980) Continuous or nocturnal oxygen therapy in hypoxemic chronic obstructive lung disease: a clinical trial. Nocturnal Oxygen Therapy Trial Group. Ann Intern Med 93:391-398
2. Medical Research Council Working Party (1981) Long-term domiciliary oxygen therapy in chronic hypoxic cor pulmonale complicating chronic bronchitis and emphysema. Lancet 1:681-686
3. Donahoe M, Rogers RM, Wilson DO, Pennock BE (1989) Oxygen consumption of the respiratory muscles in normal and in malnourished patients with chronic obstructive pulmonary disease. Am Rev Respir Dis 140:383-391
4. Skwarski K, MacNee W, Wraith PK, Sliwinski P, Zielinski J (1991) Predictors of survival in patients with chronic obstructive pulmonary disease treated with long-term oxygen therapy. Chest 100:1522-1527
5. Cooper CB, Waterhouse J, Howard P (1987) Twelve-year clinical study of patients with hypoxic cor pulmonale given long-term domiciliary oxygen therapy. Thorax 42:105-110
6. Neff TA, Petty TL (1978) Long-term continuous oxygen therapy in chronic airway obstruction. Ann Intern Med 72:621-625
7. Meyrick B, Reid L (1978) The effect of continued hypoxia on rat pulmonary arterial circulation: an ultrastructural study. Lab Invest 38:188-200
8. Hasleton PS, Haeth D, Brewer DB (1968) Hypertensive pulmonary vascular disease in states of chronic hypoxia. J Pathol 95:431-40
9. Burrows B, Niden AH, Fletcher CM, et al. (1964) Clinical types of chronic obstructive lung diseases in London and Chicago. Am Rev Resp Dis 90:14-27
10. Weitzenblum E, Hirth C, Ducolone A, et al. (1981) Prognostic value of pulmonary artery pressure in chronic obstructive pulmonary disease. Thorax 36:752-758
11. Bishop JM, Cross KW (1984) Physiological variables and mortality in patients with various categories of chronic respiratory disease. Bull Eur Physiopathol Respir 20:495-500
12. Levine BE, Bigelow DB, Hamstra RD, et al. (1967) The role of long-term continous oxygen administration in patients with chronic airway obstruction with hypoxemia. Ann Intern Med 66:639-650
13. Abraham AS, Cole RB, Bishop JM (1969) Reversal of pulmonary hypertension by prolonged oxygen administration to patients with chronic bronchitis. Circ Res 23:147-157
14. Stark RD, Finnegan P, Bishop JM (1972) Daily requirement of oxygen to reverse pulmonary hypertension in patients with chronic bronchitis. Br Med J 3:724-728
15. Gluskowski J, Jedzejewska-Makowska M, Hawrylkiewicz I, et al. (1983) Effects of prolonged oxygen therapy on pulmonary hypertension and blood viscosity in patients with adavanced cor pulmonale. Respiration 44:177-183
16. Stark RD, Finnegan P, Bishop JM (1973) Long-term domiciliary oxygen in chronic bronchitis with pulmonary hypertension. Br Med J 3:467-470
17. Cooper CB, Waterhouse J, Howard P (1987) Twelve year clinical study of patients with hypoxic cor pulmonale given long-term domiciliary oxygen therapy. Thorax 42:105-110
18. Timms RM, Khaja FV, Williams GW, et al. (1985) Hemodynamic response to oxygen therapy in chronic obstructive pulmonary disease. Ann Intern Med 102:29-36
19. Zielinski J, Tobiasz M, Hawrylkiewics I, et al. (1998) Effects of long-term oxygen therapy on pulmonary hemodynamics in COPD patients. Chest 113:65-70
20. Magee F, Wright JL, Wiggs BR, et al. (1988) Pulmonary vascular structure and function in chronic obstructive pulmonary disease. Thorax 43:183-189
21. Meyrick B, Reid L (1980) Endothelial and subintimal changes in rat hilar pulmonary artery during recovery from hypoxia: a quantitative and ultrastructural study. Lab Invest 42:603-615
22. Erelel M, Cuhadaroglu C, Ece T, Arseven O (2002) The frequency of deep venous thrombosis and pulmonary embolus in acute exacerbations of chronic obstructive pulmonary disease. Respir Med 96:515-518
23. Keller CA, Naunheim KS, Osterloh J, Espirtu J, McDonald JW, Ramos RR (1997) Histopathologic diagnosis made in lung tissue resected from patients with severe emphysema undergoing lung volume reduction surgery. Chest 111:941-947
24. Stewart Harris CH (1959) A hospital study of congestive heart failure, with special reference to cor pulmonale. Br Med J 2:201-208
25. Zielinski J, MacNee W, Wedzicha J, et al. (1997) Causes of death in patients with COPD and chronic respiratory failure. Monaldi Arch Chest Dis 52:43-47
26. Georgopoulos D, Brochard L (1998) Ventilatory strategies in acute exacerbations of chronic obstructive pulmonary disease. Eur Resp Mon 8:12-44
27. Perrin C, El Far Y, Vandenbos F, et al. (1997) Domiciliary nasal intermittent positive pressure ven-

tilation in severe COPD: effects on lung function and quality of life. Eur Resp J 10:2835-2839

28. Groenewegen KH, Schols AMWJ, Wouters EFM (2003) Mortality and mortality related-factors after hospitalization for acute exacerbations of COPD. Chest 124:459-467

29. Dal Negro RW, Rossi A, Cerveri I (2003) The burden of COPD in Italy: results from the confronting COPD survey. Respir Med 97:S43-S50

30. White AJ, Gompertz S, Stocley RA (2003) Chronic obstructive pulmonary disease: the aetiology of exacerbation of chronic obstructive pulmonary disease. Thorax 58:73-80

31. Dal Negro RW, Visconti M, Tognella S, Pomari C, Trevisan F, Micheletto C (2002) The role of viruses during COPD exacerbation: a prevalence study by direct identification on bronchial secretions. In: Proceedings. International Meeting COPD3, Birmingham, p 3

32. Hirschmann JV (2000) Do bacteria cause exacerbation of COPD? Chest 118:193-203

33. Dal Negro RW, Micheletto C, Tognella S, Visconti M, Guerriero M, Sandri MF (2005) A two stage logistic model based on the measurement of pro-inflammatory cytokines in bronchial secretions for assessing bacterial, viral, and non-infectious origin of COPD exacerbations. Journal of Chronic Obstructive Pulmonary Disease 2:7-16

34. JA Wedzicha (2002) Exacerbations, etiology and pathophysiologic mechanisms. Chest 121:136S-141S

35. Dal Negro RW, Visconti M, Tognella S, Micheletto C, Pomari C, Trevisan F (2002) Cytokine profile in sputum from non-infective exacerbation of COPD and non-atopic asthma. Eur Resp J 20(suppl 38):252S

36. Micheletto C, Pomari C, Dal Negro R (1994) Acute infections during LTOT. In: Proceedings. Highlights in Pneumology, Naples, p 44

37. Douglas NJ, White DP, Pickett CK, Weil JV, Zwillich CW (1982) Respiration during sleep in normal man. Thorax 37:840-844

38. Berthon-Jones M, Sullivan CE (1982) Ventilatory and arousal responses to hypoxia in sleeping humans. Am Rev Respir Dis 126:758-762

39. Levi-Valensi P, Weitzenbblum E, Rida Z (1992) Sleep-related oxygen desaturation and daytime pulmonary haemodynamics in COPD patients. Eur Resp J 5:301-307

40. Krop HD, Block AJ, Cohen E (1973) Neuropsychologic effects of continuous oxygen therapy in chronic obstructive pulmonary disease. Chest 64:317-322

41. Grant I, Heaton RK, Mcsweeny AJ, Adams KM, Timms RM (1982) Neuropsychologic findings in hypoxemic chronic obstructive pulmonary disease. Arch Intern Med 142:1470-1476

42. Prigatano GP, Parsons OA, Wright E, Levin DC, Hawryluk G (1983) Neuropsychologic test performance in mildly hypoxemic patients with chronic obstructive pulmonary disease. J Consult Clin Psychol 51:108-116

43. Gibson GE, Shimada M, Blass JP (1978) Alterations in acetylcholine synthesis and in cyclic nucleotides in mild cerebral hypoxia. J Neurochem 31:757-760

44. Decramer M, Gosselink R, Troosters T, Verschueren M, Evers G (1997) Muscle weakness is related to utilization of health care resources in COPD patients. Eur Respir J 10:417-423

45. Chailleaux E, Laaban JP, Veale D (2003) Prognostic value of nutritional depletion in patients with COPD treated by long-term oxygen therapy. Chest 123:1460-1466

46. Cano NJM, Roth H, Court-Fortune I, et al. (2002) Nutritional depletion in patients on long-term oxygen therapy and/or home mechanical ventilation. Eur Resp J 20:30-37

47. Petty TL, Stanford RE, Neff TA (1971) Continuous oxygen therapy in chronic airway obstruction. Observations on possible oxygen toxicity and survival. Ann Intern Med 75:361-167

48. Bone RC, Pierce AK, Johnson RL Jr (1978) Controlled oxygen administration in acute respiratory failure in chronic obstructive pulmonary disease: a reappraisal. Am J Med 65:896-902

49. West GA, Primeau P (1983) Nonmedical hazards of long-term oxygen therapy. Respir Care 28:906-912

LTOT Outcomes: Patient's and Doctor's Perspectives

S. Tognella

Since the introduction of oxygen as a therapeutic agent many years ago, much has been learnt regarding the detrimental effects of hypoxaemia and the beneficial impact of oxygen therapy on reversing hypoxaemia's complications in patients with advanced lung disease. Nowadays, oxygen is regarded as an effective prescription drug for hypoxaemic patients and long-term oxygen therapy (LTOT) has emerged as one treatment that clearly increases the length and quality of life in patients with advanced stable chronic obstructive pulmonary disease (COPD) and chronic hypoxaemia. This statement is based upon a large body of work that began in the mid-1960s and was firmly established by two major controlled clinical trials in COPD patients: the Nocturnal Oxygen Therapy Trial (NOTT) and the British Medical Research Council (MRC) [1, 2]. Successively, LTOT has been used also for respiratory failure caused by other pulmonary diseases, such as kyphoscoliosis, lung fibrosis and pulmonary embolism. Nevertheless, our experience (Fig. 1) also shows that COPD remains the major cause of chronic hypoxia requiring LTOT.

Nowadays, the large numbers of patients receiving supplemental oxygen as treatment and the high costs incurred in providing oxygen therapy necessitate the practitioner to be knowledgeable about the real effects of LTOT.

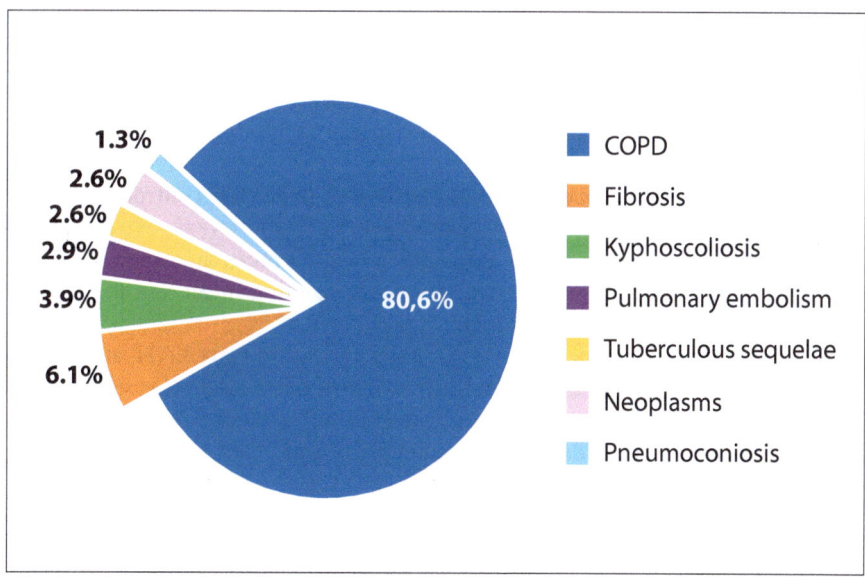

Fig. 1. Conditions justifying LTOT in the last ten years (1995-2004, n=309)

Effect of Long-Term Oxygen Therapy on Mortality

The two landmark studies, NOTT and MRC [1, 2], have clearly shown that LTOT improves survival in patients with severe COPD associated with resting hypoxaemia. In both of these studies it was shown that the more continuous the therapy, the better the survival rate.

The precise mechanism by which LTOT improves survival is not yet well understood, but is possible that it improves various haemodynamic variables.

Nevertheless, more recent clinical studies have indicated a higher mortality than that shown in earlier studies, especially in male subjects [3]. MacNee found that patients with more severe COPD may not derive a significant benefit from LTOT [4] and Soler et al. described how hypoxaemic patients with COPD treated with LTOT seem to have the same life expectancy as non-hypoxaemic patients with COPD [5].

In a 10-year ANTADIR analysis (ANTADIR, Association Nationale pour le Traitement à Domicile de l'Insuffisance Respiratoire Chronique), the mean survival for patients with chronic bronchitis was 3 years, while survival rates are slightly better for patients with bronchiectasis and asthma and worse for those with emphysema [6]. Patients with kyphoscoliosis and neuromuscular disease have the longest survival, while patients with tuberculous sequelae experience the same survival as COPD patients (3 years). Prognosis is the worst in patients with pneumoconiosis or fibrosis: 50% of these patients die during the year following the beginning of home treatment. The association of an obstructive lung disease worsens the prognosis of patients with kyphoscoliosis or neuromuscular disease and tends to bring the survival rate of the patients with pneumoconiosis or fibrosis closer to that of COPD patients. In COPD, male sex, older age, lower body mass index (BMI), FEV1 % predicted, PaO_2, and $PaCO_2$ are independent negative prognostic factors. For tuberculous sequelae and kyphoscoliosis, female sex, younger age, a high BMI, PaO_2, and $PaCO_2$ (and for kyphoscoliosis a higher FEV1/vital capacity [VC] ratio) are all independent favorable prognostic factors. In pulmonary fibrosis, lower PaO_2 and $PaCO_2$ values, a lower VC % predicted, and a higher FEV1/VC ratio are negative prognostic factors [6].

As previously reported in this book, the experience of our group involves many LTOT patients followed over twenty years. These patients have been managed with a specific home care protocol including continuous telemetric control of O_2 saturation, heart frequency and oxygen consumption [7]. We have recently analysed the last ten years of work: of 309 patients, the overall mean age when the LTOT started was 70.7 years ± 13.7 SD and the corresponding mean age when LTOT ended was 76.8 years ± 7.7 SD (Fig. 2).

Fig. 3 shows that females (30.4% of subjects) usually start LTOT almost two years later than males, and that mean life duration of LTOT subjects is shorter than expected for both males and females of the general population in Italy (National Statistics Institute - ISTAT data). LTOT males prove much closer to the ISTAT value in term of mean life duration.

Overall, mean duration of telemetric LTOT is 3.6 years ± 2.8 SD, range 0.12-13 years. Table 1 highlights that subjects with kyphoscoliosis represent the youngest group of LTOT subjects (p<0.01), starting LTOT much earlier than all other sub-

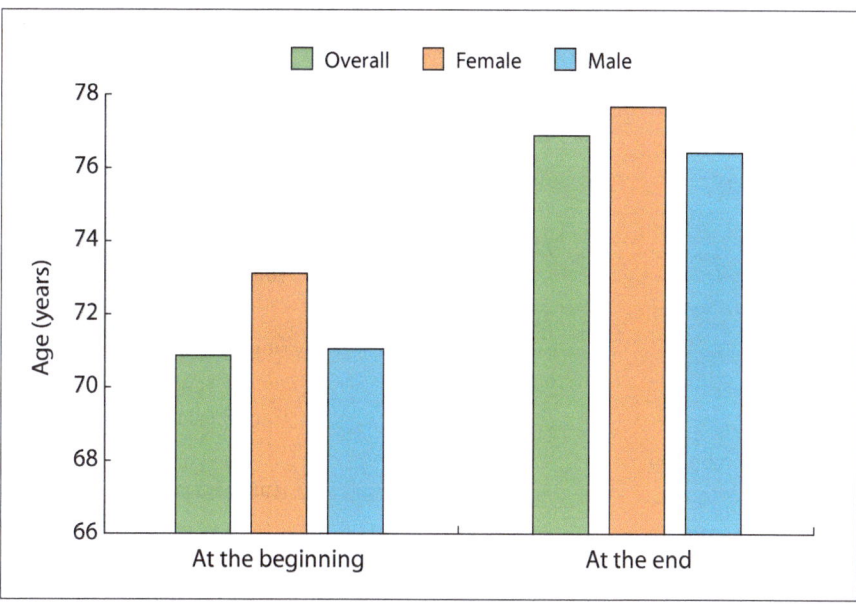

Fig. 2. Overall patients' mean age upon admission to the telemetric LTOT program and at the end of LTOT; the latter value corresponds to the patients' mean age at death in more than 98% of cases. Also reported the corresponding mean ages for males and females (n=309)

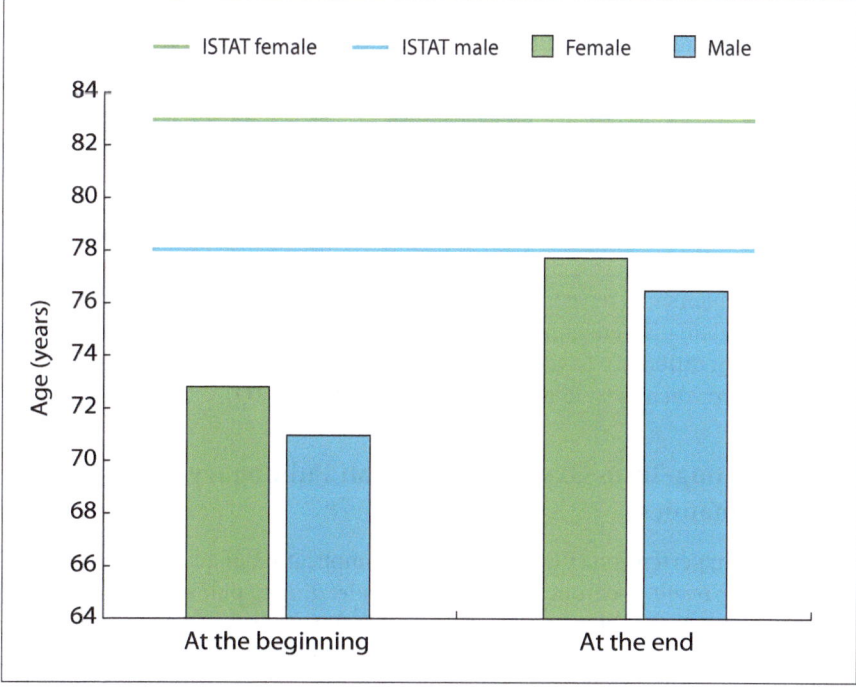

Fig. 3. Comparison of males' and females' mean ages at the beginning and at the end of telemetric LTOT compared with the corresponding mean life duration in Italy (ISTAT) (n=309)

Table 1. Mean duration of telemetric home monitoring, comparing the different causes of LTOT (n=309)

	Age at the beginning (mean ± SD)	LTOT duration (mean ± SD)
Overall	70.7 ys ± 13.7	3.6 ys ± 2.8 (min. 0.2, max. 13)
COPD	72.34 ys ± 8.5	3.6 ys ± 2.8 (min. 0.2, max. 13)
Fibrosis	71.9 ys ± 10.1	2.0 ys ± 2.0 (min. 0.4, max. 6.4)
Kyphoscoliosis	59.2 ys ± 10.2	4.7 ys ± 0.9 (min. 3.6, max. 5.4)
Pulmonary embolism	74.1 ys ± 6.9	4.0 ys ± 1.7 (min. 1.2, max. 6)
Tuberculous sequelae	72.2 ys ± 8.4	1.5 ys ± 0.6 (min. 0.9, max. 2.4)
Neoplasms	68.5 ys ± 5.2	3.2 ys ± 2 (min. 1.3, max. 6.8)
Pneumoconiosis	74.6 ys ± 3.1	3.2 ys ± 2 (min. 1.4, max. 4.6)

jects and showing the longest duration on the telemetric LTOT program.

The first positive net result of telemetric LTOT is also emphasised by considering that in the last decade of home management of severe respiratory patients, the number of survivals is progressively increasing, with more new admissions to the LTOT program than the corresponding number of LTOT interruptions (>98% due to the patients death) (Fig. 4).

While the benefits of LTOT for patients with COPD associated with hypoxaemia <60 mmHg at rest are well known, it has not been clearly established whether supplemental oxygen therapy for patients with COPD with mild-to-moderate hypoxaemia is beneficial [8-10]. Some studies [11, 12] found that there was no significant difference in the survival rates of patients with COPD with mild-to-moderate hypoxaemia (>56 mmHg) with and without LTOT.

Effect of Long-Term Oxygen Therapy on Pulmonary Haemodynamics

Pulmonary hypertension (PH) is a common complication of advanced COPD, that develops as a result of chronic alveolar hypoxia leading to pulmonary arterial wall remodelling [13, 14]. The first trials using LTOT for severe COPD patients also assessed its effects on pulmonary arterial pressure (PAP) with very encouraging results. In the MRC study [1], patients treated with oxygen for 15 hours per day showed stabilisation of PAP during almost two years of treatment, while in the

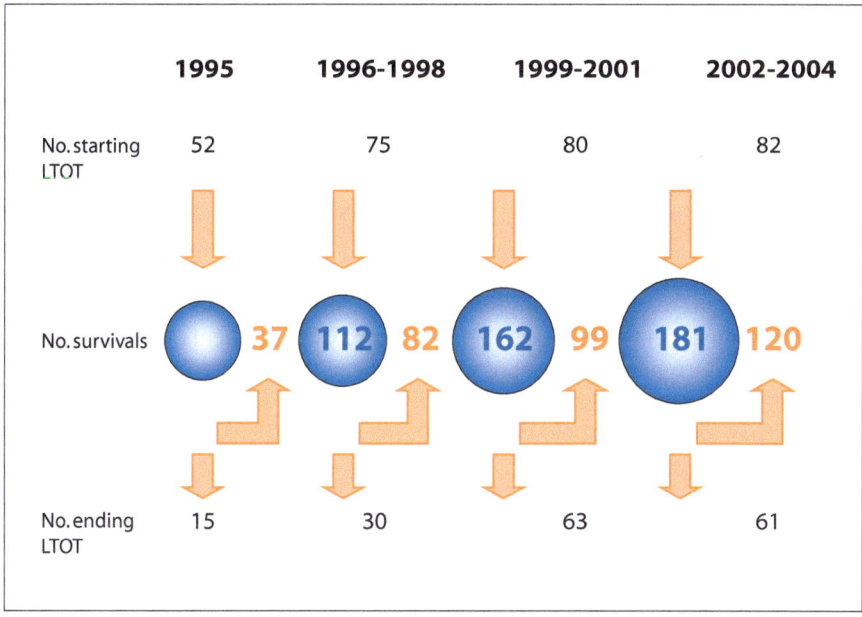

Fig. 4. Dynamic change in the number of survivals with telemetric LTOT patients in the last decade (1995-2004, n=309)

control group without oxygen therapy, PAP increased by 2.8 mmHg per year. In the NOTT trial [2], patients treated with continuous oxygen (18 hours per day) demonstrated a fall in PAP of 3 mmHg, whereas no change in PAP was observed in patients receiving oxygen for 12 hours.

Weitzenblum et al. [15] studied pulmonary haemodynamics in COPD patients before and after introduction of LTOT. Before LTOT, oxygen PAP increased on average by 1.5 mmHg per year. In the same group of patients, after introduction of LTOT (16 hours per day), PAP decreased by 2.2 mmHg per year.

More recently, Zielinski et al. [16] performed a 6-year perspective of pulmonary haemodynamics in COPD patients. The study concluded that LTOT for 14 to 15 hours per day resulted in a small reduction in pulmonary hypertension after the first two years, followed by a return to initial values and subsequent stabilisation of PAP over six years. The long-term stabilisation of pulmonary hypertension occurred despite progression of the airflow limitation and of hypoxaemia.

Cor pulmonale is defined as hypertrophy, dilation, or dysfunction of the right ventricle (RV) due to pulmonary hypertension resulting from disorders and diseases of the respiratory system. Cor pulmonale is common and accounts for approximately 80 000 deaths every year in the United States. It may result from one of numerous heterogeneous processes, all of which lead to a common clinical picture. Of these processes, COPD accounts for the great majority of cases [17].

The goals of treatment of cor pulmonale include alleviating symptoms of right heart failure, improving functional capacity, and improving survival. These goals can be achieved with correction of the major operative pathophysiologic mechanisms: hypoxaemia, acidaemia, increased pulmonary vascular resistance, and neurohormonal activation.

The goal of oxygen therapy is to relieve tissue hypoxia and to reduce the level of hypoxic pulmonary vasoconstriction, which has been shown to increase the duration of survival in patients with cor pulmonale [1, 2]. Oxygen therapy should be considered as a primary means of reducing RV afterload in hypoxaemic patients with cor pulmonale. In addition, oxygen therapy relieves renal vasoconstriction and improves oxygen delivery to critical organs, including the heart and brain [18].

One of the beneficial effects of oxygen therapy is the elimination of alveolar hypoxia, thus preventing the progression of PH and development of clinical signs of cor pulmonale. In the 1950s, a great number of COPD patients were dying from right heart failure, but the advent of LTOT changed this picture. In fact, in a recent multicenter study only 13% of COPD patients undergoing LTOT died from right heart failure, while most of patients died from chronic progressive, acute or chronic respiratory failure [19].

Effect of Long-Term Oxygen Therapy on Sleep

Recent American Thoracic Society guidelines [20] for diagnosis and treatment of COPD recommended increasing oxygen flow by 1 l/min during sleep in patients undergoing LTOT, in order to prevent nocturnal oxygen desaturation. This phenomenon is more frequent in "blue bloater" patients.

There are several mechanisms that may be responsible for nocturnal desaturations in patients with COPD. The minute ventilation decreases during sleep similarly in both normal subjects and COPD patients. The majority of desaturations appear during rapid eye movement sleep. Irregular breathing, especially shallow rapid breathing that increases physiologic dead space ventilation, and hypoventilation are responsible for these desaturations [21]. The decreased activity of intercostal muscles and the increase of upper and lower airway resistance additionally decreases alveolar ventilation. Resetting of respiratory control to higher $PaCO_2$ and lower PaO_2 during sleep also reduces ventilatory response to blood gas disorders [22].

The absence of a cough reflex during sleep in patients with disturbed mucociliary clearance increases the ventilation/perfusion imbalance due to mucous retention in the small airways. Hypoventilation and the increase of the ventilation/perfusion ratio results in transient hypoxaemic episodes, mainly during REM sleep [23].

The clinical importance of nocturnal desaturation in COPD patients is still under debate. Fletcher and coworkers found that about 25% of COPD patients with daytime PaO_2 >60 mmHg experienced nocturnal desaturation [24]. Desaturators had higher PAP at rest and during exercise [25]. During a 3-year follow-up period, desaturators treated with oxygen during sleep showed a decrease in PAP, contrary to desaturating control patients in whom PAP increased [26] and who also had a shorter survival rate [27].

However, a paper by Chaouat et al. [28] did not confirm that nocturnal desaturations in COPD patients with diurnal PaO_2 >55 mmHg resulted in a permanent increase of PAP. Generally, it was found that the level of PaO_2 during the day correlates well with nocturnal desaturations [29]. However, there are large individual variations in nocturnal hypoxaemia in COPD patients. Plywaczewski's data [30] confirm that it is rather difficult to predict nocturnal desaturations from spirometric indexes and from the diurnal PaO_2. The best predictor of nocturnal desaturation was diurnal $PaCO_2$.

In summary, around half of COPD patients undergoing LTOT experience nocturnal hypoxaemia even though they are breathing oxygen at a flow that ensures satisfactory oxygenation during the day. Desaturation during sleep may be expected in patients with a $PaCO_2$ of >45 mmHg and a PaO_2 of <65 mmHg while breathing oxygen.

Sleep-related oxygen desaturation may also be present in patients not qualifying for conventional LTOT, i.e. in patients with a diurnal PaO_2 of >55-60 mmHg [31]. Nocturnal oxygen therapy (NOT) could be justified if isolated nocturnal hypoxaemia had deleterious effects on life expectancy, which has not been convincingly demonstrated [32] or on pulmonary haemodynamics, which is rather controversial. The results of two initial studies [33, 34], suggesting an increased risk of developing pulmonary hypertension in nocturnal desaturators, without marked daytime hypoxaemia, have not been confirmed in a more recent study [35], which included a larger group of patients. This study showed that NOT given to COPD patients not filling the criteria to justify conventional LTOT, but exhibiting sleep-related oxygen desaturation, did not alter the evolution of pulmonary haemodynamics. The most relevant result of this study was the absence of significant changes in pulmonary haemodynamics in either group [35]. Authors concluded that the prescription of NOT in isolation is probably not justified in chronic obstructive pulmonary disease patients.

Effect of Long-Term Oxygen Therapy on Exercise Performance

It has been demonstrated that supplemental oxygen during exercise results in acute improvements in exercise tolerance and dyspnoea in some patients with COPD with mild hypoxaemia at rest [36, 37]. However, it has not been clarified in which type of patients with COPD such acute improvement in exercise tolerance and dyspnoea is more prominent. Moreover, it is difficult to predict the patients in which oxygen inhalation will be effective or more prominent [36, 38].

It has been suggested that mechanisms leading to improvement in exercise tolerance as a result of supplemental oxygen are multi-factorial. These factors include relief of dyspnoea, prevention of desaturation during exercise, improvement in pulmonary haemodynamics, reduction of ventilation and associated dynamic hyperinflation, and improved oxygen delivery and oxidative metabolism in respiratory and peripheral muscles during exercise [38-40].

Woodcock et al. [36] demonstrated that oxygen inhalation resulted in an increase in the 6-minute walking test by 12% and improved dyspnoea by 16% in pink puffer patients. However, in this study there was no significant correlation between the degree of these improvements and the findings from pulmonary function tests or arterial blood gas analysis at rest.

Fujimoto et al. confirmed that oxygen inhalation significantly increased the exercise performance of patients with COPD who showed mild hypoxaemia at rest [41]. In this study the improvement in exercise performance with oxygen was more prominent in the moderate-to-severe groups than in the mild group, and correlated negatively with %FEV1 predicted, but was not associated with PaO_2 at rest or the degree of desaturation during the walking test. Fujimoto's study suggests that oxygen inhalation results in greater improvement in exercise performance in patients with COPD who have severe airflow obstruction, even though these patients may show mild hypoxaemia at rest or during exercise.

It has been demonstrated that supplemental oxygen results in acute improvements in exercise tolerance and breathlessness in patients with COPD who show exercise hypoxaemia [42], but this phenomenon has not been sufficiently examined in patients without exercise hypoxaemia.

Somfay et al. [43] recently demonstrated that supplemental oxygen significantly reduces dyspnoea scores, dynamic hyperinflation assessed from inspiratory capacity maneuver results, ventilation, and respiratory frequency during exercise also in nonhypoxaemic patients with severe COPD. This improvement in exercise capacity was found to correlate with a reduction in dynamic hyperinflation. Dynamic hyperinflation, which readily develops in patients with COPD with severe airflow obstruction and hyperinflation, has a deleterious mechanical effect on the respiratory muscles, contributing to a sensation of breathlessness, and limits exercise capacity [44]. It is therefore not surprising that the effect of oxygen was most prominent in patients with severe airflow obstruction. This suggests that the improvement in exercise capacity and dyspnoea is a result of supplying oxygen for patients with severe airflow obstruction, and that mild hypoxaemia may be primarily related to reduced dynamic hyperinflation caused by the decrease in augmented ventilation during exercise.

Effect of Long-Term Oxygen Therapy on Cognitive-Neurological Dysfunction and on Quality of Life

Patients with severe COPD suffer from cognitive impairment, anxiety and depression, more than in the control population. Thus many factors, not only social and physical, but also patients' expectations and their hopes and fears may contribute to impaired health status in patients with severe COPD. Exercise dyspnoea may increase anxiety of patients and lead to loss of control over their disease. It has been shown that although 50% of the variance in a disease-specific quality of life questionnaire can be explained by cough, wheeze, walking distance, and anxiety, that still left 50% of the variance in the health score attributable to other factors [45]. The reason for the psychological dysfunction in patients with chronic hypoxaemia is largely unknown. It is unlikely that direct effects of hypoxia on brain metabolism are important; some action on brain neurotransmitters, coupled with the effects of aging in this population, are more probable [45].

It is very difficult to evaluate the possible relationship between neuropsychiatric impairment and LTOT. There are data from the NOTT trial that show improvement in neuropsychiatric function, which seems to be better in the continuous oxygen group than the nocturnal oxygen group, especially at the 12-month mark [46]. There are no other well-controlled trials addressing this; however, in reviewing a number of studies using historical or case controls, it was found that LTOT did not necessarily improve neuropsychiatric scores, although oxygen may have stabilised these symptoms [47].

Several studies have shown that quality of life (QoL) is impaired in patients with COPD and hypoxaemia [48, 49]. Furthermore, in patients with moderate-to-severe hypoxaemia, the QoL score is related to the degree of hypoxaemia when measured using a disease-specific questionnaire [50]. However, few studies have addressed the impact of LTOT on QoL, and available results are conflicting. In an ancillary study to the NOTT trial, there was no improvement in QoL over six months in patients with hypoxic COPD treated with oxygen compared to age-matched controls without COPD [51]. Okubadejo [52] and other investigators have reported similar results [53, 54], detecting no change in the QoL of patients with COPD after six months of LTOT. Conversely, there are some reports of improved QoL after LTOT [55, 56].

QoL can also be impaired by erectile impotence, that is commonly encountered in male patients with respiratory failure and hypoxia. In the Aasebo study, 42% of the patients experienced reversal of sexual impotence during LTOT: responders showed a significant increase in arterial PaO_2 and serum testosterone, and a decline in sex hormone binding globulin compared to non-responders [57].

Effect of Long-Term Oxygen Therapy on Hospitalisation

Since the cost of home oxygen therapy is high, demonstration of any economical advantage from a reduction in hospitalisation related to use of LTOT is important. An early study from the 1970s and two recent studies, all including a small number of patients acting as their own control, have indicated that LTOT decreases hospitalisations [58, 59]. However, the MRC study, which had a randomised control group, failed to confirm this advantage of LTOT [1]. Today, it is considered unethical to undertake placebo-controlled studies in COPD patients with chronic hypoxaemia. Conversely, studies with patients acting as their own control may be biased by the fact that frequent hospitalisations and the decision to prescribe LTOT are interrelated: physicians may be more likely to initiate LTOT in patients with frequent hospitalisations rather than in patients with a stable condition. A reduction in hospitalisations after initiation of LTOT could therefore simply reflect a "regression to the mean phenomenon", a bias that has not been focussed on in previous studies [58, 59]. Taking this into account, the effect of LTOT on hospitalisations, in a larger study with patients acting as their own control, was investigated by Ringbaek [60]. In addition, given that not all patients use oxygen for the recommended number of hours (at least 15 daily), the authors investigated whether compliance with hours spent on oxygen had an impact on hospitalisation. Authors concluded that in hypoxaemic COPD patients LTOT is associated with a reduction in days spent in hospital and that the beneficial effect of LTOT on hospitalisation seems to reflect an effect of therapy *per se* and not a "regression to the mean phenomenon" [60]. Similar data were found also by our group: by analysing the year before LTOT and the three following years of active telemetric LTOT, a substantial drop in hospital admissions was seen, particularly for COPD versus fibrotic patients (Fig. 5). Nevertheless, in fibrotic patients the total number of in-days did not drop significantly. These peculiar trends seem to suggest that, even though some admissions can be avoided during LTOT also in fibrotic patients, when the clinical condition precipitates an unavoidable hospitalisation, the duration of the hospital stay cannot be reduced because, unfortunately, the patient is proceeding towards the lung's "end stage".

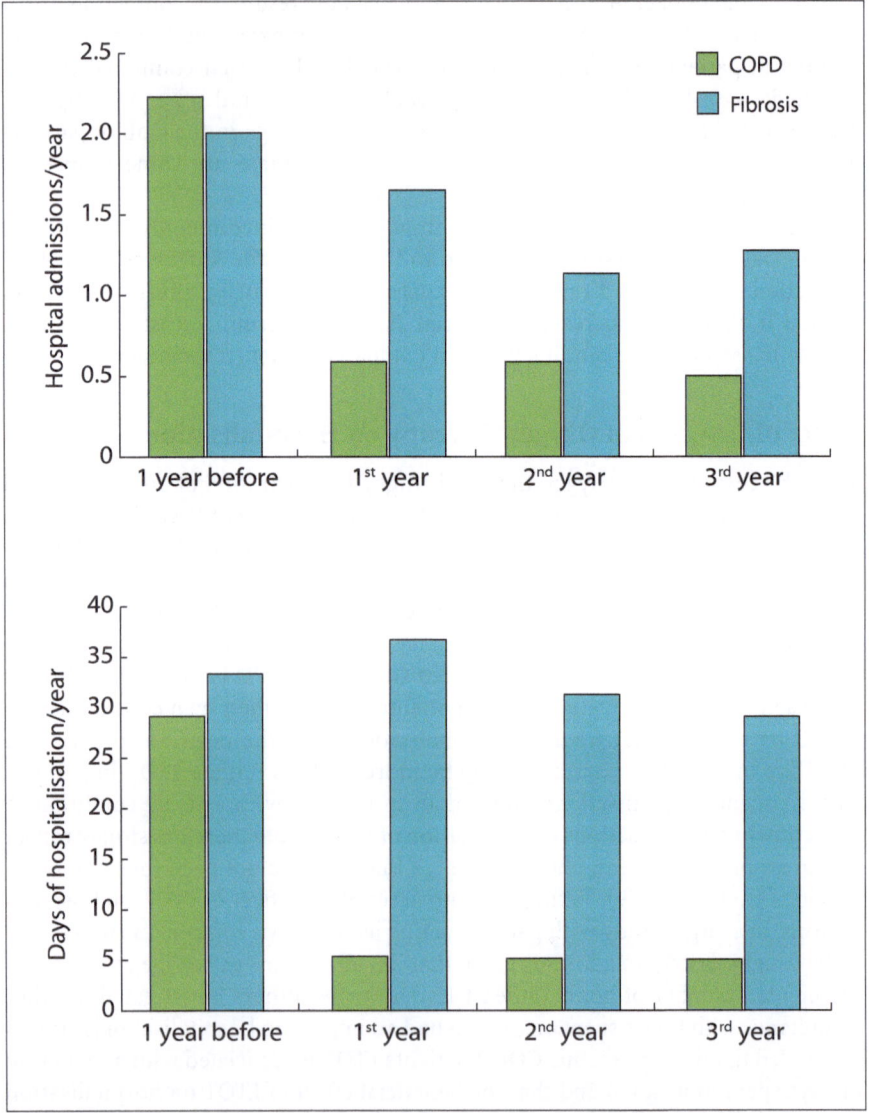

Fig. 5. Frequency and duration of hospitalisation before LTOT and during three years of active telemetric LTOT

Effect of Long-Term Oxygen Therapy on Nutritional Status

An association between malnutrition, weight loss and mortality has been demonstrated in patients with COPD, but the prognostic influence of malnutrition has not been exhaustively evaluated in patients with the most severe COPD treated with LTOT. Toth et al. suggest that nutritional status is closely linked with prognosis in patients with chronic respiratory insufficiency treated with domiciliary LTOT: low BMI, low plasma cholesterol and low albumin are related to worse 2-year survival in such patients [61]. Chailleux's study shows that nutritional depletion defined by a low BMI was associated with increased mortality and hospitalisation rates, independent of the severity of airway obstruction in a large population of hypoxaemic patients with COPD treated with home LTOT. In this study, the highest survival and lowest hospitalisation rates were observed in obese patients [62]. This surprising finding has been confirmed by other Authors [63-65] despite the fact that obesity is usually associated with an increased mortality that mainly results from an increased cardiovascular risk. There is no clear pathogenic mechanism that could explain why obesity should improve the survival of patients with severe COPD. It has been suggested that obese patients with COPD are better protected from a decrease in body cell mass during periods of acute illness because of higher energy reserves [64]. Another hypothesis is that obesity in itself contributes to low FEV1, so that obese patients with COPD classified as having severe COPD may in fact have a less severe airflow obstruction and therefore longer survival [66].

In conclusion, LTOT is the only intervention known to increase life expectancy in patients with lung disease. It also improves quality of life, especially when used in conjunction with pulmonary rehabilitation. Specific benefits include amelioration of cor pulmonale, enhanced cardiac function, increased body weight, reversal of polycythaemia, improved neuropsychiatric function and exercise performance, reduced pulmonary hypertension, improved skeletal-muscle metabolism, and possible reversal of sexual impotence. In addition, use of ambulatory oxygen therapy reduces the need for hospitalisation.

References

1. Report of the Medical Research Council Working Party (1981) Long-term domiciliary oxygen therapy in chronic cor pulmonale complicating chronic bronchitis and emphysema. Lancet 1:681-685
2. Nocturnal Oxygen Therapy Trial Group (1980) Continuous or nocturnal oxygen therapy in hypoxemic chronic obstructive lung disease: a clinical trial. Ann Intern Med 93:391-398
3. Crockett AJ, Cranston JM, Moss JR, Alpers JH (2001) Survival on long-term oxygen therapy in chronic airflow limitation: from evidence to outcomes in the routine clinical setting. Intern Med J 31(8):448-454
4. MacNee W (1992) Predictors of survival in patients treated with long-term oxygen therapy. Respiration 59(Suppl 2):5-7
5. Soler M, Michel F, Perruchoud AP (1991) Long-term oxygen therapy for cor pulmonale in patients with chronic obstructive pulmonary disease. Respiration 58(Suppl 1):52-56
6. Chailleux E, Fauroux B, Binet F, et al. (1996) Predictors of survival in patients receiving domiciliary oxygen therapy or mechanical ventilation. A 10-year analysis of ANTADIR observatory. Chest 109:741-749
7. Dal Negro RW (2000) Long-term oxygen tele-home monitoring, the Italian perspective. Chest 2000 Companion Book. pp 247-249

8. Zielinski J (1998) Long-term oxygen therapy in COPD patients with moderate hypoxaemia: does it add years to life? Eur Respir J 12:756-758
9. Calverley PM (2000) Supplementary oxygen therapy in COPD: is it really useful? Thorax 55:537-553
10. McDonald, CF, Blyth, CM, Lazarus, MD, et al. (1995) Exertional oxygen of limited benefit in patients with chronic obstructive pulmonary disease and mild hypoxaemia. Am J Respir Crit Care Med 152:1616-1619
11. Gorecka D, Gorzelak K, Sliwinski P, et al. (1997) Effect of long-term oxygen therapy on survival in patients with chronic obstructive pulmonary disease with moderate hypoxaemia. Thorax 52:674-679
12. Veale D, Chailleux E, Taytard A, et al. (1998) Characteristics and survival of patients prescribed long-term oxygen therapy outside prescription guidelines. Eur Respir J 12:780-784
13. Meyrick B, Reid L (1978) The effect of continued hypoxia on rat pulmonary arterial circulation. An ultrastructural study. Lab Invest 38(2):188-200
14. Hasleton PS, Heath D, Brewer DB (1968) Hypertensive pulmonary vascular disease in states of chronic hypoxia. J Pathol Bacteriol 95(2):431-440
15. Weitzenblum E, Sautegeau A, Ehrhart M, Mammosser M, Pelletier A (1985) Long-term oxygen therapy can reverse the progression of pulmonary hypertension in patients with chronic obstructive pulmonary disease. Am Rev Respir Dis 131(4):493-498
16. Zielinski J, Tobiasz M, Hawrylkiewicz I, Sliwinski P, Palasiewicz G (1998) Effects of long-term oxygen therapy on pulmonary hemodynamics in COPD patients: a 6-year prospective study. Chest 113(1):65-70
17. Murphy ML (1989) Chronic cor pulmonale. Dis Mon 35:653-718
18. Reihman DH, et al. (1985) Effect of hypoxaemia on sodium and water excretion in chronic obstructive lung disease. Am J Med 78:87-94
19. Zielinski J, MacNee W, Wedzicha J, et al. (1997) Causes of death in patients with COPD and chronic respiratory failure. Monaldi Arch Chest Dis 52(1):43-47
20. American Thoracic Society (1995) Standards for the diagnosis and care of patients with chronic obstructive pulmonary disease. Am J Respir Crit Care Med 152:S77-S121
21. Hudgel DW, Martin RJ, Capehart M, et al. (1983) Contribution of hypoventilation to sleep oxygen desaturation in chronic obstructive pulmonary disease. J Appl Physiol 55:669-677
22. Douglas NJ, White DP, Veil JV, et al. (1982) Hypercapnic ventilatory response in sleeping adults. Am Rev Respir Dis 126:758-762
23. Mulloy E, McNicholas WT (1996) Ventilation and gas exchange during sleep and exercise in severe COPD. Chest 109:387-394
24. Fletcher EC, Miller J, Devine J, et al. (1987) Nocturnal oxyhemoglobin desaturation in COPD patients with arterial oxygen tensions above 60 mmHg. Chest 92:604-608
25. Fletcher EC, Luckett RA, Miller T, et al. (1989) Exercise hemodynamics and gas exchange in patients with chronic obstructive pulmonary disease, sleep desaturation and daytime PaO_2 above 60 mmHg. Am Rev Respir Dis 140:1237-1245
26. Fletcher EC, Luckett RA, Goodnight-White S, et al. (1992) A double-blind trial of nocturnal supplemental oxygen for sleep desaturation in patients with chronic obstructive pulmonary disease and daytime PaO_2 above 60 mmHg. Am Rev Respir Dis 145:1070-1076
27. Fletcher EC, Donner CF, Midgren B, et al. (1992) Survival in COPD patients with daytime PaO_2 >60 mmHg with or without nocturnal oxygen desaturation. Chest 101:649-655
28. Chaouat A, Weitzenblum E, Kessler R, et al. (1997) Sleep related O_2 desaturation and daytime pulmonary hemodynamics in COPD patients with mild hypoxaemia. Eur Respir J 10:1730-1735
29. McKeon JL, Murre-Allan K, Saunders NA (1988) Prediction of oxygenation during sleep in patients with chronic obstructive lung disease. Thorax 43:312-317
30. Plywaczewski R, Sliwinski P, Nowinski A, et al. (2000) Incidence of nocturnal desaturation while breathing oxygen in COPD patients undergoing long-term oxygen therapy. Chest 117:679-683
31. Fletcher EC, Miller J, Divine GW, Fletcher JG, Miller T (1987) Nocturnal oxyhemoglobin desaturation in COPD patients with arterial oxygen tensions above 60 Torr. Chest 92:604-608
32. Fletcher CE, Donner C, Midgren B, et al. (1992) Survival in COPD patients with a daytime PaO_2 >60 mmHg with and without nocturnal oxyhemoglobin desaturation. Chest 101:649-655
33. Fletcher EC, Luckett RA, Miller T, Costarangos C, Kutka N, Fletcher JG (1989) Pulmonary vascular hemodynamics in chronic lung disease patients with and without oxyhemoglobin desaturation during sleep. Chest 95:757-764
34. Levi-Valensi P, Weitzenblum E, Rida Z, et al. (1992) Sleep-related oxygen desaturation and daytime pulmonary haemodynamics in COPD patients. Eur Respir J 5:301-307
35. Chaouat A, Weitzenblum E, Kessler R, et al. (1997) Sleep-related O_2 desaturation and daytime pulmonary haemodynamics in COPD patients with mild hypoxaemia. Eur Respir J 10:1730-1735
36. Woodcock AA, Gross ER, Geddes DM (1981) Oxygen relieves breathlessness in "pink puffers."

Lancet 1:907-909
37. Dean NC, Brown JK, Himelman RB, et al. (1992) Oxygen may improve dyspnea and endurance in patients with chronic obstructive pulmonary disease and only mild hypoxaemia. Am Rev Respir Dis 146:941-945
38. O'Donnell DE, Bain DJ, Webb KA (1997) Factors contributing to relief of exertional breathlessness during hypcroxia in chronic airflow limitation. Am J Respir Crit Care Med 155:530-535
39. O'Donnell DE, Lam M, Webb KA (1998) Measurement of symptoms, lung hyperinflation, and endurance during exercise in chronic obstructive pulmonary disease. Am J Respir Crit Care Med 158:1557-1565
40. Garrod R, Paul EA, Wedzicha JA (2000) Supplemental oxygen during pulmonary rehabilitation in patients with COPD with exercise hypoxaemia. Thorax 55:539-543
41. Fujimoto K, Matsuzawa Y, Yamaguchi S, Koizumi T, Kubo K (2002) Benefits of oxygen on exercise performance and pulmonary hemodynamics in patients with COPD with mild hypoxemia. Chest 122:457-463
42. Ries AL, Carlin BW, Carlin V, et al. (1997) Pulmonary rehabilitation: joint ACCP/AACVPR evidence-based guidelines. J Cardiopulm Rehabil 17:371-405
43. Somfay A, Porszasz J, Lee SM, et al. (2001) Dose-response effect of oxygen on hyperinflation and exercise endurance in nonhypoxaemic COPD patients. Eur Respir J 18:77-84
44. O'Donnell DE, Webb KA (1993) Exertional breathlessness in patients with chronic airflow limitation: the role of lung hyperinflation. Am Rev Respir Dis 148:1351-1357
45. Wedzicha JA (2000) Effects of LTOT on neuropsychiatric function and quality of life. Respir Care 45(1):119-124
46. Petty TL, Nett LM (1983) The history of long-term oxygen therapy. Respir Care 28(7):859-865
47. MacIntyre NR (2000) Long-term oxygen therapy: conference summary. Respir Care 45(2):237-245
48. McSweeney AJ, Grant I, Heaton RK, Adams KM, Timms RM (1982) Life quality of patients with chronic obstructive pulmonary disease. Arch Intern Med 142:473-478
49. Guyatt G, Townsend M, Berman L, Pugsley S (1987) Quality of life in patients with chronic airflow limitation. Br J Dis Chest 81:45-54
50. Okubadejo AA, Jones PW, Wedzicha JA (1996) Quality of life in patients with chronic obstructive pulmonary disease and severe hypoxaemia. Thorax 51:44-47
51. Heaton RK, Grant I, McSweeney AJ, et al. (1983) Psychologic effects of continuous and nocturnal oxygen therapy in hypoxemic chronic obstructive pulmonary disease. Arch Intern Med 143: 1941-1947
52. Okubadejo AA, Paul EA, Jones PW, et al. (1996) Does long-term oxygen therapy affect quality of life in patients with chronic obstructive pulmonary disease and severe hypoxaemia? Eur Respir J 9:2335-2339
53. Heaton RK, Grant I, McSweeney AJ, et al. (1983) Psychologic effects of continuous and nocturnal oxygen therapy in hypoxemic chronic obstructive pulmonary disease. Arch Intern Med 143:1941-1947
54. Lahdensuo A, Ojanen M, Ahonen A, et al. (1989) Psychosocial effects of continuous oxygen therapy in hypoxemic chronic obstructive pulmonary disease patients. Eur Respir J 2:977-980
55. Dilworth JP, Higgs CMB, Jones PA, et al. (1990) Acceptability of oxygen concentrators: the patient's view. Br J Gen Pract 40:415-417
56. Eaton T, Lewis C, Young P, Kennedy Y, Garrett JE, Kolbe J (2004) Long-term oxygen therapy improves health-related quality of life. Respir Med 98(4):285-93
57. Aasebo U, Gyltnes A, Bremnes RM, Aakvaag A, Slordal L (1993) Reversal of sexual impotence in male patients with chronic obstructive pulmonary disease and hypoxemia with long-term oxygen therapy. J Steroid Biochem Mol Biol 46(6):799-803
58. Crockett AJ, Moss JR, Cranston JM, Alpers JH (1993) The effect of home oxygen therapy on hospital admission rates in chronic obstructive airways disease. Monaldi Arch Chest Dis 48:445-446
59. Buyse B, Demedts M (1995) Long-term oxygen therapy with concentrators and liquid oxygen. Acta Clin Belg 50:149-157
60. Ringbaek TJ, Viskum K, Lange P (2002) Does long-term oxygen therapy reduce hospitalisation in hypoxaemic chronic obstructive pulmonary disease? Eur Respir J 20:38-42
61. Toth S, Tkacova R, Matula P, Stubna J (2004) Nutritional depletion in relation to mortality in patients with chronic respiratory insufficiency treated with long-term oxygen therapy. Wien Klin Wochenschr 116(17-18):617-621
62. Chailleux E, Laaban JP, Veale D (2003) Prognostic value of nutritional depletion in patients with COPD treated by long-term oxygen therapy: data from the ANTADIR observatory. Chest 123(5):1460-1466
63. Wilson DO, Rogers RM, Wright EC, et al. (1989) Body weight in chronic obstructive pulmonary disease: The National Institutes of Health Intermittent Positive-Pressure Breathing Trial. Am Rev Respir Dis 139:1435-1438

64. Gray-Donald K, Gibbons L, Shapiro SH, et al. (1996) Nutritional status and mortality in chronic obstructive pulmonary disease. Am J Respir Crit Care Med 153:961-966
65. Schols AM, Slangen J, Volovics L, et al. (1998) Weight loss is a reversible factor in the prognosis of chronic obstructive pulmonary disease. Am J Respir Crit Care Med 157:1791-1797
66. Landbo C, Prescott E, Lange P, et al. (1999) Prognostic value of nutritional status in chronic obstructive pulmonary disease. Am J Respir Crit Care Med 160:1856-1861

Telemedicine for Home-Ventilated Patients

E.E. Guffanti, D. Colombo, A. Fumagalli, C. Misuraca, A. Viganò

Mechanical Ventilation

The modern era of mechanical ventilation began during the poliomyelitis epidemics in the middle of the 20th century when non-invasive negative pressure ventilation by iron lung was essentially the only weapon available. The realisation that negative pressure ventilation was not enough to beat poliomyelitis induced the search for other types of ventilation, resulting in development of the modern positive pressure ventilator and the use of positive pressure ventilation by tracheotomy. The era of invasive ventilation led to a reduction in mortality from polio. One of the consequences of this victory was the development of a population of survivors dependent upon prolonged life-sustaining technology, who had no option but to remain in hospital for an indefinite time. Many operators, from doctors to the engineers, worked with patients and their families to find new technological and organisational solutions. The staff discovered that positive pressure ventilation by mouthpiece or lip-seal permitted a safe non-invasive ventilation without needing negative pressure devices and without the need for a tracheotomy. At first, non-invasive positive pressure ventilation for home use was applied to patients with hypoventilation due to neuromuscular diseases, central control of breathing disorders and skeletal deformities. In recent years, there has been a growing interest in the use of non-invasive ventilation due to the increasing incidence of respiratory insufficiency caused by lung diseases [1].

At the same time, a smaller group of patients affected by respiratory insufficiency underwent tracheotomy and were ventilated 24 hours a day. Many of them, due to clinical problems, were judged unweanable. Discharge from hospital to home of this population of patients leads to different types of problems. Home mechanical ventilation requires not only a medical prescription written by an expert physician, but also a correct and exact initial clinical assessment, an evaluation of home environment, home-care documentation of organisation and a complete and accurate education of the patient, and when possible, of the family. All these problems are even more complex in patients ventilated continuously by tracheotomy.

If patients and their families are appropriately selected and trained, the application of long-term home ventilation can reduce the time spent in hospital, increase their feeling of security, improve their quality of life and reduce the costs for the health organisation. This is even more evident with innovative use of telemedicine techniques.

Telemedicine and Ventilation at Home

Telemedicine is defined as the use of information and communication technology to provide health care services to individuals who are distant from the health care provider [2]. Therefore, telemedicine could be considered an umbrella term that encompasses any medical activity involving an element of distance and in which a doctor—patient interaction involves telecommunication [3].

Many articles report the feasibility of various applications of telemedicine, but only a few of them report a controlled comparison of a telemedicine application to conventional means of providing health services. The same can be said for cost effectiveness studies of telemedicine interventions [4, 5].

Roine and coworkers [2] analysed more than 1000 papers and concluded that the most convincing published evidence, regarding the effectiveness of telemedicine, deals with teleradiology, teleneurosurgery, telepsychiatry, transmission of echocardiographic images and the use of electronic referrals enabling e-mail consultations and video conferencing between primary and secondary health care providers.

Promising results have been obtained for the transmission of electrocardiograms and teledermatology.

If we consider the application of telemedicine in respiratory diseases, only a few articles have been published and it is interesting to note that in a recent analysis performed in UK, not one of 216 telemedicine projects was dedicated to respiratory diseases [6].

Telemedicine has been employed in chronic obstructive pulmonary disease (COPD) patients, in patients receiving long-term oxygen therapy, in asthma patients and also in lung transplant recipients to allow the early detection of acute infection and rejection of the allograft [7-10].

Finkelstein and coworkers [11] applied telehomecare to a group of patients affected by COPD or by chronic heart failure (CHF): virtual visits increased patient satisfaction and quality of the home care programs.

Maiolo et al. [12] investigated the feasibility of telemonitoring services for patients with severe respiratory illness and long-term oxygen therapy. The patients were monitored at home for 12 months, during which time determination of arterial oxygen saturation and heart rate were performed twice a week and automatically transmitted to the hospital's processing centre via a normal telephone line. The results showed a reduction of acute exacerbations and of hospital admissions during the telemonitoring phase.

A Japanese group of investigators published a paper about telemedicine support systems in the home care of patients with chronic respiratory failure. They concluded that the telemedicine network system has the potential to improve clinical outcomes and to provide home care services to patients affected by chronic respiratory illness [13]. Other Authors investigated the cost effectiveness of telemedicine applied to respiratory disease [14-16].

In 2004, the results of a questionnaire were published, in which 2380 Italian pneumologists evaluated telemedicine in respiratory practice in Italy. Thirty-nine projects were reported, only six of which involved ventilators: no information is available about parameters monitored in these studies [17].

What is it Useful to Monitor?

Many non-invasive home-ventilated patients utilise the ventilator only during the night while others are ventilated for some hours during the day as well. Patients who have undergone invasive ventilation by tracheotomy often have 24 hour ventilation. These different types of patients have different monitoring needs.

The pneumologist must appropriately select patients on the basis of their clinical needs, their clinical history and home environment. After taking into consideration these factors, the relevant parameters to monitor must be decided upon, whether it be just oxygen saturation and heart rate or also ventilator parameters.

On the basis of the clinical status at the moment of discharge, the pneumologist must draw up a plan for home organisation and must agree with the practioner on the timing of the telematic check that will differ depending on whether the patient needs invasive or non-invasive ventilation. Furthermore, the physician must decide what type of recording he wishes to analyse, whether it be whole nocturnal recordings or occasional data recorded during the day. Before discharge from hospital, the patient and his caregiver must be fully trained in the use of the chosen monitoring system and the way in which to transmit data.

Systems of Monitoring

Simple pulseoxymeters, able to trasfer recorded data by normal telephone line, can be utilised to monitor heart rate and oxygen saturation. Many commercial devices are available that are capable of transmitting the recorded data. When the physician decides to monitor ventilator parameters as well, different types of devices can be used.

Sally

This is a modular multiparametric digital recorder able to acquire and memorise different clinical data non-invasively, including: arterial oxygen saturation and heart rate; liquid oxygen level of a cryogenic system for oxygen therapy; data derived from other external devices (i.e. spirometers, ECG, capnometers, ventilator, blood pressure gauge).

For data coming from ventilators, the record of the different parameters is obtained by measuring the pressure and the air flow into the ventilator circuit via specific sensors. In particular, for ventilator data the device works with a specific VTN-A module. This is adaptable to each type of ventilator, connecting with the transducer to the ventilator circuit. It can measure some variables directly and calculate other variables (e.g., PEEP, I/E ratio, respiratory rate, minute ventilation, maximal inspiratory pressure). Furthermore, the module is able to measure data with different levels of accuracy, including:

- Volumes: from 100 to 300 ml +/-20%; from 300 to 2000 ml +/-10%
- Flows : +/-2200 ml/sec +/-10%
- Pressures: +/-350 cm H_2O +/-2%
- Time: +/-20 ms

The memorised data can be transmitted via the Internet to a hospital's processing centre for analysis. Sally is able to activate a questionnaire option via which the physician can receive and store clinical information about the patient. Oxygen saturation, heart rate and other data coming from external devices are memorised by the digital recorder. Sally has memory capacity of 4 MB and is able to record data over 24 hours. Moreover, there is the possibility to extend the memory with a MMC/SD (MultiMedia Card/Secure Digital) if needed. The data are saved and are transmitted to the central server by integrated modem so they can be analysed via the Internet by any common browser. The safety of the transmission is guaranteed by a high level system of cryptography based on 128 bit keys.

Oxytel

Oxytel is a multiparametric digital recorder with an integrated pulseoxymeter. It is a multichannel recorder able to receive and save data from external devices such as pulmonar ventilators, capnometers, spirometers, oxygen vessels and other devices able to transmit analogical/digital signals. The recorded information can be sent automatically and on demand.

Oxytel is integrated with a pulseoxymeter provided by Nellcor, which can record and save saturimetric data and patient pulse rate using different protocols. The Oxytel software works perfectly in a Windows environment, allowing the physician to visualise and process all acquired data in an easy, fast and correct way.

Oxytel is also equipped with a special function called "Questionnaire". This option permits the physician to receive and save information from personalised questions directly sent to the patient and answered with either "yes" or "no". The data can be transmitted to a central server by integrated modem so they can be analysed via the Internet by the physician.

ALS Con-Tel II

This is a multiparametric system to monitor subjects suffering from respiratory insufficiency. The recorder has a Nellcor integrated pulseoxymeter able to contemporarily control up to four medical devices, to acquire data to transmit to a dedicated Web portal (ALS Gate). This receives and elaborates data, permitting analysis by the physician. The data are transferred from the patient's house to portal Web by normal telephone line. ALS Con-Tel II can record noninvasively oxygen saturation and heart rate, and receive and save the data coming from any medical device able to connect with it. The instrument has some integrated devices, including a capnograph NPB 70 Tyco/Oridion, ECG 12 leads Cardiette, Spirometer Cosmed, Blood Pressure gauge Bp One OPCB cardiette, pulmonar ventilators and oxygen cylinder Freelox II. As with the other systems, Con-Tel II also has the questionnaire option that permits the physician to receive information through personalised questions directly sent to the patient. Using a personal password on the Internet, both the physician and the general practitioner can observe and analyse the data of their patient. ALS Con-Tel II utilises security protocols and a system of cryptography to defend the privacy of the patient's data.

Our Experience

The Rationale

Since 1989 our Respiratory Unit has been treating patients affected by respiratory insufficiency. More than 400 patients have been ventilated in hospital and then at home. Now we follow more than 270 ventilated patients at home, many of whom are invasively ventilated by tracheotomy, sometimes up to 24 hours a day (Fig. 1, Table 1).

All these ventilated patients need special care, especially when they are discharged from hospital. If the patients are ventilated for more than 16 hours a day and are tracheotomised, the physician must draw up an accurate home organisation plan paying particular attention to the safety and emergency aspects. The patients must have two ventilators, the caregivers must be trained in tracheoaspiration, management of tracheotomy and of ventilator accessories (e.g., humidifier, ventilator circuit and filters).

Problems are encountered when the practitioners and nurses are inexperienced with these conditions. For these reasons, patient discharge always results in a vast range of medical, ethical, legal and social problems.

At the end of 1998 we began to think about how to resolve some of these difficulties and, being stimulated by the experience of cardiologists of our Institute in the telemetric management of patients with CHF, we tried to develop a specific system to remotely monitor invasively ventilated patients.

We decided to utilise a new system, more complete and complex in respect to the traditional and known devices for monitoring oxygen saturation and heart rate. In fact, we needed not only to verify real-time oxygen saturation, heart rate, respiratory rate and all the respiratory parameters deriving from continuous ventilation but we also wanted to have the possibility of directly modifying these parameters remotely, from our Respiratory Unit.

By an unrestricted grant of a home care company (HCC) (Gastec-MEDICAIR), an informatic engineer developed dedicated software to enable remote monitor-

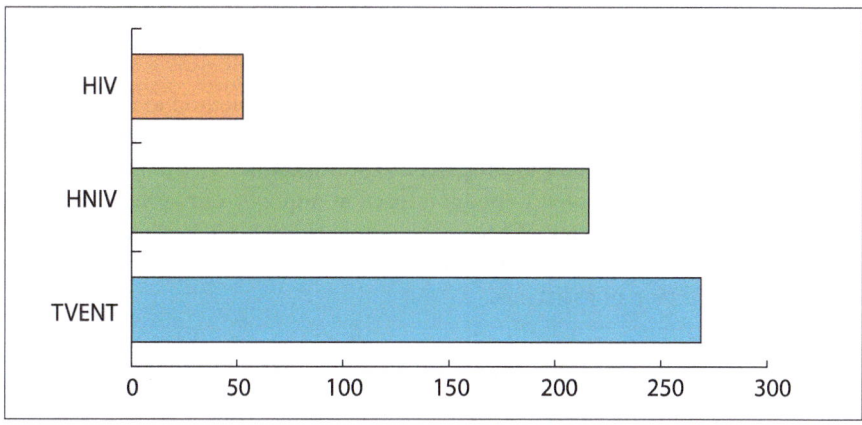

Fig. 1. Home-ventilated population followed by our Respiratory Unit at the end of 2004. HIV, home invasively ventilated patients (n=53); HNIV: home non-invasively ventilated patients (n=216); TVENT, total of ventilated patients

Table 1. Gender, age, diagnosis and daily period of ventilation of telemonitored patients

Patient	Sex	Age	Diagnosis	Ventilation hours
MM	F	75	ALS	24
MA	M	72	Encephalopathy	24
MA	F	74	Post-TBC	12
GM	M	74	COPD	14
CI	F	63	ALS	24
SA	M	66	CHF	24
LD	M	25	DMD	24
RG	M	80	COPD	14
SR	M	81	COPD	14
CA	M	72	ALS	24
CG	M	76	ALS	24

ALS, amyotrophic lateral sclerosis; DMD, Duchenne muscular dystrophy

ing and modification of the ventilator parameters. For more than two years the new software has been checked daily in our Unit, with particular regard to efficacy and safety. Our first goal was to be sure that there was a perfect and on-line correspondence between the changes set out by central computer in the Unit and those carried out by ventilator of the patient. The second goal was to defend the privacy of the transmitted data. Furthermore, the system has an audio-video connection to permit the patients and their families to see and to talk with the operators in our Unit and vice versa. In June 2001, in agreement with the Health Agency of Lecco and with the HCC, we discharged the first connected patient, a woman suffering from ALS and ventilated by tracheotomy 24 hours a day.

After this experience, we connected ten other patients. All of them were invasively ventilated by tracheotomy: seven were ventilated continuously and four were ventilated for 12-14 hours a day.

All the families were informed of the aims of this new method to monitor ventilated patients, with particular regard to the possibility of modifying the ventilator parameters by a computer located in our control centre. All patients and their families except two consented to be monitored at home by our system. In agreement with the Health Agency of Lecco, the Public Home Care Service assisted all the patients in agreement with the general practitioner and with our Unit, on the basis of a shared plan of assistance.

Characteristics of the New System

The interactivity of the system we have developed has been achieved by using communication devices in the patient's home and in the control centre located in our hospital's semi-intensive Respiratory Unit.

Patient's Home

The devices available at home are the following:
- BREAS ventilator type PV403
- NONIN pulseoxymeter
- ECG acquisition device with serial interface
- Home Care Unit (UHC) serial concentrator
- POTS line modem or GSM radio modem
- TV set with SCART interface
- TV camera with modem and TV interface

Medical data is acquired through the serial interfaces of the specific MDD devices, selected for the presence of a standard interface and the openness of the transmission protocol. Some manufactures required a non-disclosure agreement before releasing the communication protocol and interface to the development team. The Home Care Unit (UHC) is a MDD compliant communication device specially developed to provide a stable and safe interface with the local devices, and able to collect specific data from the ventilator, the pulseoxymeter and the ECG unit. It can answer an incoming modem call and establish a packet-oriented cryptographically-protected bidirectional communication with the remote control unit. According to device protocols, the UHC can, if so instructed from the remote control centre, switch devices on or off, change settings, start or stop acquiring data and restore a safe and stable state in case of communication failure. The hardware is based on a 8 bit microcontroller with 256 KB of ROM program memory and 128 KB data RAM programmed completely in C language. The software was developed *ad hoc* for the specific interfaced devices and was completely developed in house, without reference to an external operating system.

Input/output interfaces are electrically isolated to keep patient and medical devices safe. User interface is, by design, very simple. A small number of LEDs signal normal working status with a green light, keeping the whole system almost "invisible" to the patient. We used a standard line modem to connect to the available phone line or a GSM modem phone where a land line was not available.

Control Centre

- PC standard with Windows operating systems (98 and above) with color CRT
- Line modem or GSM modem
- MEDICAIR software for remote UHC control
- TV set with SCART interface
- TV camera with modem and TV interface

User interface is Windows-based due to the low cost of commercial systems and the basic operator training required, i.e. "point and click" interactions. The graphic power of commercially available hardware allows the development of a pleasant interface, almost reconstructing the visual feeling of the remote device, obtaining an intuitive and simple usage procedure. The remote control software MEDICAIR is developed in C language and works using two separate processes on the same machine: the presentation process and the communication process.

The presentation process is graphically oriented and implements the user interface, authenticates the user ID and password, allows the selection of a remote patient using a preloaded drop-down list and draws in a split screen a graphical "virtual keyboard" of the remote ventilator with "clickable" buttons emulating the real keys on the machine. On the left side of the screen the received information of oxygen saturation, heart rate and ventilator are displayed in real time and provide a continuous recording. It is possible to acquire an ECG strip of a few seconds and show the 2 ECG traces full screen. Users, after identification, are only authorised to start a connection and visualise the remote status of the devices. Activating a "doctor mode" with the proper ID and password, the software allows special commands to be sent to the remote ventilator to change the working parameters selected using the virtual keyboard or a fast multi-setting screen. All activity is logged to a permanent file for usage control and medical traceability and responsability.

The communication process is a separate process without a user interface, operating at a higher priority and security level, and acting as a "middle-man" between the user interface and the remote device. This separate process implements connecting, coding/decoding and the remote identification procedure and is specifically coded to be resistant to all typical communication problems like noise, unexpected line drops and local or remote power outages. It is also safe from the "hang ups" at the presentation level that often occur in the Windows environment. Full control of the local communication device (line modem or GSM modem), the paired authorisation process between the server and the remote client, the local logging of the activity and many other protection techniques grant a safe and protected communication channel for the commands coming from the presentation process and also act as synchronising buffers to and from the remote device.

In addition, all these techniques are proven in the field to be resistant to "third party" attack or intrusion, providing highly reliable and traceable communication between the units. As a last safety measure, the system can be activated only if a security USB dongle is connected to the PC server. This HW dongle can act also as an identification and serialisation unit, avoiding not only any unauthorised activity, but also working as server ID, allowing connection only to specifically identified and "paired" remote units.

Evolution of the Experience

Different protocols of monitoring were used to follow each patient. Two types of contact between the Central Unit and the patient's home were planned. The first included both computer and audio-video connection, the second only the former. With only audio-video connection, the operator at Central Unit could observe the trend of ventilator parameters relative to the patient's ventilated 24 hours. He could call the family whenever he observed significant or dangerous changes in these parameters, alerted by visual red signals.

The computer connection took place every day for the first week after discharge. Later this check was performed once a week, if patient conditions were stable. The complete connection was periodically activated by the Central Unit and whenever the caregiver called the centre, depending on the problem. Any contact with the connected patient is recorded by the computer software, including the name of the specialist in charge, the data, the time and parameter changes.

Each MD in our Unit can access the monitored patients' file. The MD must enter his personal password to access all the data. If the alarms or parameters need to be changed he must retype his personal password and after that the software allows modifications to be carried out. Every change of parameter must be confirmed by the specific command "apply changes" and at any moment the MD can return to the original setting of the ventilator using the command "restore the parameters". The computer allows the MD to observe the entire trends of ventilation parameters, oxygen saturation and heart rate during the changes. By audio-video connection the MD watches the patient and can speak with the caregiver.

Only on ten occasions we needed to change the original ventilation parameters. These changes applied to seven of the eleven patients. Two patients, in spite of parameter resetting needed to be taken to the hospital by emergency services staff. Following are the specific cases.

GM (COPD) was recovering in ICU from respiratory failure due to pneumonia; he stayed in the ICU for 4 days and then went home. Six months later GM died in the ICU of abdominal occlusion.

CG (ALS) was in the ICU for only two days after an angina attack and returned again due to angina. He was taken to the Hospital Emergency Ward where he stayed for 24 hours.

MA, who is currently still alive, has returned to our Unit three times during monitoring. This patient is the only one monitored mostly for social reasons: she lives alone. The cause of the three hospital admissions was always an acute exacerbation of COPD that could have been treated at home if there had been the help of a trained caregiver.

During four years of monitoring, eight patients died for different reasons and after different periods of active monitoring, as detailed in Table 2.

Four patients died due to their illnesses. ALS and encephalopathy are progressive and the patients died after a long period of illness. In particular, CI died ten years after the diagnosis of ALS and nine years after invasive ventilation. In 1995 this patient, tracheotomised one month previously in the ICU, was discharged for the first time from our Respiratory Unit, on continuous ventilation.

The patient SA, affected by CHF, died suddenly three months after discharge from the hospital. He was ventilated continuously. This type of monitoring permitted the patient to live the last three months of his life at home.

The patient LD, suffering from DMD, was 25 years old, and had already surpassed the average life expectancy. He stayed in our hospital for seven months after a tracheotomy performed in the ICU. He was ventilated continuously and our monitoring system allowed him to be transferred to the Nursing Facility, which was located near his home. He died suddenly due to fatal arrhythmia without developing any respiratory problems.

GM, suffering from COPD, died in the ICU after an acute abdominal occlusion.

Table 2. Diagnosis, monitoring length and cause of death in our telemonitored patients

Patient	Sex	Diagnosis	Period of monitoring	Months	Cause of death
MM	F	ALS	6/2001-4/2004	34	ALS
MA	M	Encephalopathy	9/2001-2/2004	29	Encephalopathy
MA	F	Post-TBC	1/2002-alive		
GM	M	COPD	10/2001- 8/2003	22	Abd. occlusion
CI	F	ALS	2/2002-12/2004	34	ALS
SA	M	CHF	8/2001-11/2001	3	Arrhythmia
LD	M	DMD	9/2003-10/2003	2	Arrhythmia
RG	M	COPD	5/2004-2/2005	9	CerVas accident
SR	M	COPD	7/2004-alive		
CA	M	ALS	3/2005-alive		
CG	M	ALS	8/2001-3/2005	42	ALS

RG died at home by cerebrovascular accident: he was affected by both COPD and lung cancer. In the last month he was not able to walk and he had to be ventilated for more than 14 hours a day.

Limits and Advantages of the System

After 4 years of experience, we can clearly evaluate our monitoring system.

Limits

No Control Group
It is very difficult to have fair controls in this situation. Using a similar group of patients to verify if monitoring is representing a real advantage would not be a correct comparison, since external factors are too many and too important not to be considered. Even if we take for granted that COPD and ALS had the same evolution in each patient, many other elements can interfere with the efficacy of the treatment. The social and economic situation of the patient, the availability of the family to take care of him and the organisation of assistance at the patient's home by specific nursing and medical support, all represent key variables for the determination of the evolution of pathology and its prognosis. All these factors, in fact, are connected to the frequency of readmission to the hospital, the length of hospitalisation and the use of emergency services.

Number of Connected Patients
The study was considered to be preliminary experimentation and the budget allocated was limited. No patient paid for this service. The local Health Agency organised the home care, the HCC offered all the necessary facilities and our Unit followed all patients.

Technical Limits
To control the ventilator remotely, it is necessary to be familiar with the specific software. Some companies will not provide their software. For this study, we adapted the patients to the BREAS ventilator type PV403, a model that allowed us to choose between pressometric and volumetric ventilation.

Advantages

Patients and Their Families
The system permits patients to be discharged earlier, with more certainty of safety than a normal discharge. It is obvious how the quality of life of the patients and their families improves with the patient at home rather than in the hospital. The family caregiver can have the staff of nurses and physicians that followed the patient in hospital at his disposal: he has only to connect to the Central Unit and speak with the operator. The system is based on the use of simple devices present in the patient's home, a TV set with SCART interface and a phone line.

TV camera with modem and TV interface, POTS line modem or GSM radio modem are the only devices that must be bought.

Even if in this experimental phase no patient paid for the service, we tried to keep the costs of the system as low as possible, as in the near future this experience will theoretically become a regular service.

Local Health Agencies
The efficiency of a system of telemedicine is evaluated by its capability to reduce the general cost of assistance. The expected results are the reduction of hospital admissions and of the use of emergency services during the telemonitoring period.

On the basis of our experience with this population of invasively ventilated patients, we believe that our new system of monitoring will be able to attain these results. Our patients had either no or very short hospitalisations. When contacted by caregivers alarmed by the management of some minor problems a simple monitoring of the trend of oxygen saturation and ventilation parameters is sufficient to reassure the caregivers and the patients. In this way many calls to emergency services were avoided. The improved quality of life of the patients produces more satisfaction in the family members taking care of them. This satisfaction derives not only from the well-being of the patient but also from the increased sense of certainty in management of the all relevant problems related to home invasive ventilation. The Health Agency also benefits from this family satisfaction.

Another advantage of our system is the possibility for the operators of home care organisation, for the staff of emergency services and also for the practitioner to have on-line advice about every problem, either clinical or inherent to the management of ventilator.

Physician and Respiratory Unit
As already said, at the moment of discharge the pneumologist must draw up a home organisation plan to minimise the dangers and the risks for the patient and his family. Monitoring trends of vital parameters of the patient and modifying the setting of the ventilator in function of his medical needs makes the physician more secure

in his decision to discharge the invasively ventilated subject.

From the organisation's point of view, the possibility to discharge patients earlier gives the opportunity to admit other critical patients to the Respiratory Unit. For the ICU this is a real advantage, and in terms of efficiency without decreasing efficacy, both our Unit and the whole Health System benefits.

Telemedicine in Home-Ventilated Patients: the Present and the Future

We have shown that the systems to monitor home-ventilated patients are diverse. Some are able to monitor oxygen saturation and heart rate only, others like our system are also able to monitor ventilator parameters.

On the basis of the clinical status of the patient at the moment of discharge, the pneumologist must decide if it is useful to monitor the patient remotely. In this case he must choose which system can give wider clinical benefits at the minimal cost.

Following these criteria, in the last years we began monitoring both invasively and non-invasively ventilated patients. We have selected our dedicated system, described above, to be adapted only to invasively ventilated patients.

At the same time, we are following 10 non invasively-ventilated patients by simple pulseoxymetry. These patients send their nocturnal saturimetry by phoneline to a server every 15 days. We analyse the records via the Internet and we send our answers by e-mail. Another 10 non-invasively ventilated patients are followed by our Unit, 5 with Oxytel and 5 with the Sally system.

Once a week, with different systems (see above), we analyse the nocturnal data concerning the trend of oxygen saturation and ventilator parameters.

For these 20, as for the 11 invasively ventilated patients, the monitoring is performed to reduce hospitalisations and to improve quality of life. In any case, the known systems cannot be considered as an alternative to direct home assistance by home care services. These systems, from the most simple to the most complex, are necessary to manage the ventilated patients and for this reason they become complementary to direct assistance. The monitoring systems are an important means to better assist them.

The case of MA (Table 2, patient 3) who, in spite of monitoring, has returned many times to our Respiratory Unit confirms that no significant results are possible without direct assistance.

However, our experience with invasively ventilated patients encourages the vision that hospital care at home could be achieved. The rationale is that such services increase patient satisfaction and reduce costs without adverse effects on clinical outcome.

In 2002, the Italian Health Ministry published a conclusive document about hospital care at home: respiratory diseases, in particular COPD and respiratory insufficiency, are indicated among the diseases that could benefit from home hospitalisations [18]. Even if it is very difficult to organise this form of assistance, experiences such as these should encourage clinicians to consider this form of management in patients affected by respiratory diseases [19].

Hospital care at home could be a solution for a population of survivors dependent upon ventilators who up until now have had no option but to remain in hospital for an indefinite time, often in the same ICU where the tracheotomy was performed.

Only a few Units, in fact, are able to wean from ventilators or to organise patient discharge when the patients are unweanable. These long periods of hospitalisation are incompatible with the natural needs of the disabled patients, that is, to stay at home near their families without excessive risk. Furthermore, long hospitalisations increase hospital organisational problems and management costs.

We think that our system of monitoring these patients could be useful to encourage earlier discharge of patients and to keep them at home, without decreasing the feeling of security and without increasing the real risks.

However, to be really effective our experience needs to be transferred to other situations, to enable the creation of a network between respiratory units able to treat patients who are invasively and continuously ventilated. A common call centre could receive calls from the caregiver of each single patient and put him in connection with the reference centre. In this case, the clinical data of each patient, recorded on an informatic card and using special passwords, could be available for consultation via the Internet. In this way, the network of respiratory units utilising shared protocols could monitor an elevated number of patients, optimising all the resources.

Thus, it would be possible to monitor not only the single patient but also the nursing facilities that actually do not currently follow these patients because they are afraid of not being able to manage the ventilation system. Obviously, our system must be considered as a dynamic one, and technological evolution will improve its architecture, increasing its efficacy and security.

Legal Problems

Telemedicine represents a modified medical approach with respect to usual medical procedures. In these cases it is very important to give the patients and their caregivers complete and correct information about any new methods employed. They must be informed about the risks of the method and the therapeutic alternatives. Furthermore, it is important to define the capacity of the medical staff to utilise informatic and telematic devices. Finally, it is necessary to establish the responsibility of each operator to be trained in the method and who subsequently must become an expert on ventilator devices.

References

1. Goldberg AI (2002) Noninvasive mechanical ventilation at home. Chest 121:321-324
2. Roine R, Ohinmaa A, Hailey D (2001) Assessing telemedicine: a systematic review of the literature. CMAJ 165:765-771
3. Wootton R (2001) Telemedicine. BMJ 323:557-560
4. Whitten PS, Mair FS, Haycox A, May CR, Williams TI, Hellmich S (2002) Systematic review of cost effectiveness studies of telemedicine interventions. BMJ 324:1434-1437
5. Noel HC, Vogel DC, Erdos JJ, Cornwall D, Levine F (2004) Home telehealth reduces healthcare costs. Telemed J E Health 10:170-183
6. Debnath D (2004) Activity analysis of telemedicine in the UK. Postgraduate Med J 80:335-338
7. Young M, Sparrow D, Gottlieb D (2001) A telephone-linked computer system for COPD care. Chest 119:1565-1775

8. Di Re L, Di Nicola A, Ariano C, Tomassini P (2000) Utilità del telemonitoraggio nell'ossigenoterapia a lungo termine. Rass Pat App Resp 15:294-301
9. Finkelstein J, Cabrera MR, Hripcsak G (2000) Internet-based home asthma telemonitoring. Can patients handle the tecnology? Chest 117:148-155
10. Morlion B, Knoop C, Paiva M, Estenne M (2002) Internet-based home monitoring of pulmonary function after lung transplantation. Am J Respir Crit Care Med 165:694-697
11. Finkelstein SM, Speedie SM, Demiris G, Veen M, Lundgren JM, Poth S (2004) Telehomecare: quality, perception, satisfaction. Telemed J E Health 10:122-128
12. Maiolo C, Mohamed EI, Fiorani CM, De Lorenzo A (2003) Home telemonitoring for patients with severe respiratory illness: the Italian experience. J Telemed Telecare 9:67-71
13. Koizumi T, Yamaguchi S, Hanaoka M, Fujimoto K, Kubo K, Nakai K, Takizawa M, Murase S, Kobayashi T, Suzuoka M (2003) Telemedicine support system in home care of patients with chronic respiratory failure: preliminary results. Nihon Kokyuki Gakkai Zasshi 41:173-176
14. Dal Negro R, Pomari C, Micheletto C (1995) Ossigenoterapia domiciliare a lungo termine sotto controllo telematico: aspetti farmacoeconomici. Farmacoeconomia 2:43-46
15. Shapira ZM, Make AH (2002) Cost effectiveness of telemedicine for the delivery of outpatient pulmonary care to a rural population. Telemed J E Health 8:281-291
16. Potena A (2005) Impiego clinico della telemedicina in pneumologia e rapporto costo/benefici. Rass Pat App Resp 20:3-5
17. De Tullio, Dottorini M, Quaglia A, Amaducci S, Moretti AM (2004) La telemedicina in pneumologia: i risultati di un questionario in Italia. Rass Pat App Resp 19:11-17
18. Comitato Ospedalizzazione Domiciliare (DM 12/4/2002) Documento conclusivo: Caratterizzazione dei servizi di cura domiciliare. Ministero della Salute, www.ministerosalute.it/pubblicazioni
19. Ram FS, Wedzicha JA, Wright J, Greenstone M (2004) Hospital at home for patients with acute exacerbations of chronic obstructive pulmonary disease: systematic review of evidence. BMJ 329:315

Economic Evaluation of Treating Patients with Long-Term Oxygen Therapy with or without Telemetric Monitoring

R. Ravasio, R.W. Dal Negro, C. Lucioni

Introduction

The limits on the availability of resources in the medical establishments of economically developed countries necessitates that choice of treatment be based not only on its clinical aspects but also on the economic factors of the available alternatives.

Economic evaluation studies today tend to focus primarily on high-profile technologies, only briefly considering the more specialized sectors, i.e. services with a more limited budget profile or pathologies considered "non-emotional" in the eyes of the decision makers [1].

The present evaluation is an exception since it focuses on a more specialized sector: long-term oxygen therapy (LTOT) [2, 3]. Oxygen therapy was introduced in Europe in the early 1980s specifically for the treatment of chronic obstructive pulmonary disease (COPD) and more generally for the treatment of lung pathologies [4, 5].

The aim of this study is the economic evaluation of home-based oxygen therapy, specifically in patients with telemetric monitoring compared to patients without it.

Material and Methods

The study involves data from two cohorts of patients from the Lung Department of Bussolengo Hospital (Verona): (a) 1995, patients with LTOT and telemetric monitoring and (b) 2003 (control group), patients with only LTOT. The two groups of patients were monitored for 2 years. The evaluation was in line with the National Health Service guidelines. The costs were validated for 2004.

The information obtained for both groups included patients' diagnosis and the mean number of exacerbations requiring hospitalization per year. Both groups suffered from lung pathologies, mostly COPD (89%).

For the resources used and the cost evaluation required for LTOT with or without telemetric monitoring, data from a 1995 [6] study were used, which calculated the mean daily cost of LTOT on the basis of the following factors: gas analysis, oxygen therapy, medical–nursing staff, drug treatment and telemetric monitoring. Hospitalization costs due to exacerbations were taken from a study by Lucioni et al. [7].

Results

Table 1 shows the mean annual number of hospitalizations due to exacerbations for the two groups, observed during the first 2 years of the study.

Table 1. Mean number and duration of hospitalization episodes (over a 1-year period)

Description	First year		Second year	
	With TM	Without TM	With TM	Without TM
Mean hospitalization episodes per patient	0.7	1.6	0.5	1.5
Mean length of stay (days)	11.6	21.0	7.4	20.9

TM, telemetric monitoring

The data show that both the mean number of hospital admissions per patient and the mean length of stay in hospital per visit were significantly lower in the 1995 group than the 2003 group. More specifically, a comparison of the first year shows that the 2003 group's mean annual number of hospitalizations per patient was 1.6, while for the 1995 group it was 0.7 (-56.3%). This difference increased (-66.7%) when considering data from the second year of the study (1.5 vs. 0.5).

The Cost of Home-Based Treatment

Table 2 from the study of Micheletto et al. [6] shows the original values for 1995 and the inflated values for 2004 (ISTAT index) of mean daily costs associated with a home-based oxygen therapy: gas analysis, oxygen therapy, medical–nursing staff, drug treatment and telemetric monitoring.

Table 2. Mean daily costs of LTOT (€)

Description	1995	2004
Gas analysis	0.62	1.64
O_2 (1.5 l/m in x 18 h/day)	6.66	7.39
Medical–nursing staff	1.86	2.3
Drug treatment	0.64	1.05
Telemetric monitoring	0.21	0.41

Table 3. Mean daily cost per patient with LTOT with or without telemetric monitoring (€)

Description	With TM		Without TM	
Gas analysis	1.64	12.82%	1.64	13.25%
O_2 (1.5 l/m in x 18 h/day)	7.39	57.78%	7.39	59.69%
Medical-nursing staff	2.3	17.98%	2.3	18.58%
Drug treatment	1.05	8.21%	1.05	8.48%
Telemetric monitoring	0.41	3.21%	0	0.00%
Mean daily cost	**12.79**	**100%**	**12.38**	**100%**

Based on these results, we calculated a mean daily average cost of € 12.79 per patient with telemetric LTOT and a cost of € 12.38 per patient with only LTOT (Table 3).

In both cases, the major cost (60% of the total) was the oxygen supply. The second highest cost was the medical and nursing staff (approximately 13%). The mean daily cost difference of € 0.41 (+3.3%) between the two treatments was to be found in the extra daily services required to carry out the telemetry.

The mean annual cost per patient was thus € 4,668.35 (for the 1995 group) and € 4,518.70 (for the 2003 group).

The Cost of Hospitalizations

In the study of Lucioni et al. [7], 90% of patients leaving hospital after an exacerbation (COPD) were assigned one of two disease-related groups (DRGs): either DRG 088 (chronic lung obstruction; 69%) or DRG 087 (pulmonary oedema and respiratory failure; 23.6%). The remaining hospital admissions were categorized according to one of a vast number of possible DRGs (see Table 4).

Table 4. DRG distribution

DRG Code	DRG description	n	%
088	Chronic obstructive pulmonary disease (COPD)	500	69.5%
087	Pulmonary oedema and respiratory failure	169	23.5%
475	Diagnosis related to the respiratory system and assisted respiration	13	1.8%
089	Pneumonia and pleurisy, age >17 with complications	9	1.3%
144	Diagnosis related to complication of the circulatory system	7	1.0%
Other		21	2.9%
Total		**719**	**100%**

Based on the DRG distribution and the relative reimbursement costs, the adjusted mean cost for each hospitalization episode due to a COPD exacerbation was calculated to be € 3,218 (Table 5).

Multiplying the adjusted mean cost of the DRG by the mean number of hospitalization episodes, we calculated the mean annual cost for hospitalizations both of the 1995 group and the 2003 group during the first and second year of the study (Table 6).

Table 5. Adjusted mean DRG cost (€)

Hospitalization costs according to DRG	All DRGs
n	719
Mean	3,218
Min.	601
Max.	96,398

Table 6. Mean annual cost of hospitalization episodes due to exacerbations per patient (€)

Description	First year		Second year	
	With TM	Without TM	With TM	Without TM
Hospitalization cost	2,252.60	5,148.80	1,609.00	4,827.00

Finally, we calculated the mean annual costs of treatment (LTOT and exacerbations) for the two groups of patients.

During the first study year, the group of patients with telemetric LTOT was characterized by a lower mean annual cost than the group without telemetry (-28%). This difference increased during the second study year (-33%).

This saving of € 2,746.55 in the first year and of € 3,068.35 in the second year, despite the higher average cost of the telemetric services (€ 4,668.35 vs. 4,518.70), is attributed to the lower average cost as a result of the fewer hospitalization episodes (Table 7).

Table 7. Total mean annual costs

Description	First year		Second year	
	With TM	Without TM	With TM	Without TM
LTOT costs	4,668.35	4,518.70	4,668.35	4,518.70
Hospitalization costs	2,252.60	5,148.80	1,609.00	4,827.00
Total treatment cost (mean)	6,920.95	9,667.50	6,277.35	9,345.70

Conclusion

The current economic evaluation shows that the use of telemetric monitoring with LTOT patients allows for a better control of the pathology, reducing the risk of hospitalizations due to exacerbations by 50% and leading to considerable economic savings for the National Health Service.

References

1. Mantovani L (1995) Quadro teorico di riferimento. In: Garattini L (ed) L'intervento privato in sanità. Kailash Editore, Milan
2. Garattini L, Tediosi F (2000) L'ossigeno terapia domiciliare in cinque paesi europei: un'analisi comparativa. Mecosan 35:137-148
3. Corsi F, Garattini L, Tediosi F (1999) I dispositivi medici nei principali paesi europei. Edizioni Kappadue, Milan
4. Miselli V (1995) Assistenza al paziente domiciliare. Il Pensiero Scientifico Editore, Rome
5. Rees PJ, Dudley F (1998) Oxygen therapy in chronic lung disease. Br Med J 317:871-874
6. Micheletto C, Pomari C, Righetti P, Dal Negro R (1995) A 2-year health economics survey on 61 subjects in telemetric LTOT: preliminary results (abstract). Eur Resp J 7 (Suppl 18):266
7. Lucioni C, Donner CF, De Benedetto F, et al. (2004) I costi della broncopneumopatia cronica ostruttiva in Italia. Presentazione della prima fase dello studio ICE ("Italian Costs for Exacerbations in COPD"). PharmacoEconomics (Italian research articles) 6:5-14

Continuing Quality Improvement in the Management of H-LTOT

M. Farina, S. Tognella

Quality and Its Evolution in the International Arena

Attention to Quality began in the early 1900s within the textile industry, where it was mostly linked to testing of the final product. At a later date, in addition to the quality check of the final product, a number of tests were added for the different production phases (process control); for example, testing the industrial components and materials of which the final product was made. The concept of Quality thus started off by including only the quality of the final product but then moved on to include the entire production cycle and industrial process.

Following this trend, different countries introduced conventions and norms to regulate the management of the various industrial stages. Within the medical arena, as for the industrial one, it is possible to date the origins of Quality assessment. This activity, termed "medical accreditation", has its roots in a declaration by the American College of Surgeons during the "Third Congress of North American Surgeons" in 1912.

Subsequently, other accreditation organisations emerged, for example in Canada the Canadian Council on Accreditation of Hospitals, today know as the Canadian Council of Health Facilities Accreditation, in Australia the Council on Healthcare Standards (ACHS) founded by the Australian Medical Association and the Australian Hospital Association in 1974, in the United Kingdom the Hospital Accreditation Programme (the only recognised accreditation scheme), and others in New Zealand, Argentina, France, Germany, Netherlands, Poland, Sweden and Spain.

In the American healthcare system in particular, many scientific societies followed the initial accreditation programme and its evolution: particular importance is given to the Joint Commission on Accreditation of Hospitals (JCAH), founded in 1951, which was recognised by the Federal Government in 1965 as the official accreditation system for medical structures. In 1988 the JCAH accreditation activities extended to include also health facilities other than hospitals, and thus the organisation changed its name to Joint Commission on Accreditation of Healthcare Organisations (JCAHO).

In the 1980s Donabedian's contribution proved to be crucial. He maintained that whilst respecting the individuality of each system, to bring about change in the present and future health status, the healthcare facility had to involve all the individual parts of its production system by identifying and rationalising the various sectors and roles (i.e. work environment, equipment, resources, organisation of labour etc.) and by governing all the procedures involved in the complex clinical process (such as the therapeutic and diagnostic procedure, follow-up etc).

Today, these variables are still considered the basis on which the quality of healthcare rests, especially when referring to the evaluation of established criteria and indicators within the healthcare system.

The Evolution of the Concept of Quality in Italy

In Italy in 1984 the Society for the Evaluation and Revision of the Quality of Healthcare and Medical Treatment, today known as the Italian Society for Quality in Healthcare (SIQuAs-VRQ), started raising awareness on "Continuing Quality Improvement (CQI)".

Within this arena the term "Quality" has various definitions, including:
- Based on the evaluation of citizens' problems and needs, the main aim we need to reach is to clearly identify objectives, recognise the characteristics of the most significant and important cures and define the best measures to evaluate performance and results (McMaster Health Services Research Group, Canada).
- The relationship between the health improvement actually being attained and what could be obtained on the basis of current knowledge, resource availability and patient characteristics (Donabedian).
- The level of satisfaction reached in meeting the (usually implicit) needs and expectations of clients through the inherent characteristics of the product (ISO 9000:2000).

All these definitions underline the central role of the customer-user and the importance of responsibilities, resources and organisation of the healthcare system.

For the Italian healthcare system an important role was played by decrees n. 502/92 and 517/93, the Service Chart, as well as a decree of 14 January 1997 (outlining the minimum technological and organisation requirements), and finally the more recent "Ter reform" 229/99 on accreditation. Each of these led to a number a changes which, taken together, focus the attention specifically on:
- More autonomy to single regions
- More autonomy to single organisations
- Financial incentives for performance
- The customer's role.

The accreditation concept can be summarised in the three-level structure presented in Fig. 1, from the more basic (i.e. accreditation to operate) to the highest level (i.e. accreditation for excellence). These levels are closely linked to the guidelines set out by scientific societies and their related technical standards.

The ISO 9000 norms fall within the internationally recognised Continuing Quality Improvement system with its related evaluation agencies already present in Italy. These norms, released in 1987 by the worldwide ISO (International Standardisation Organisation), have their roots in the critical analysis and integration of the different convention-norms already present in a number of different countries. These convention-norms focus on the global management tools for guaranteeing industrial quality and they are today recognised in over 100 coun-

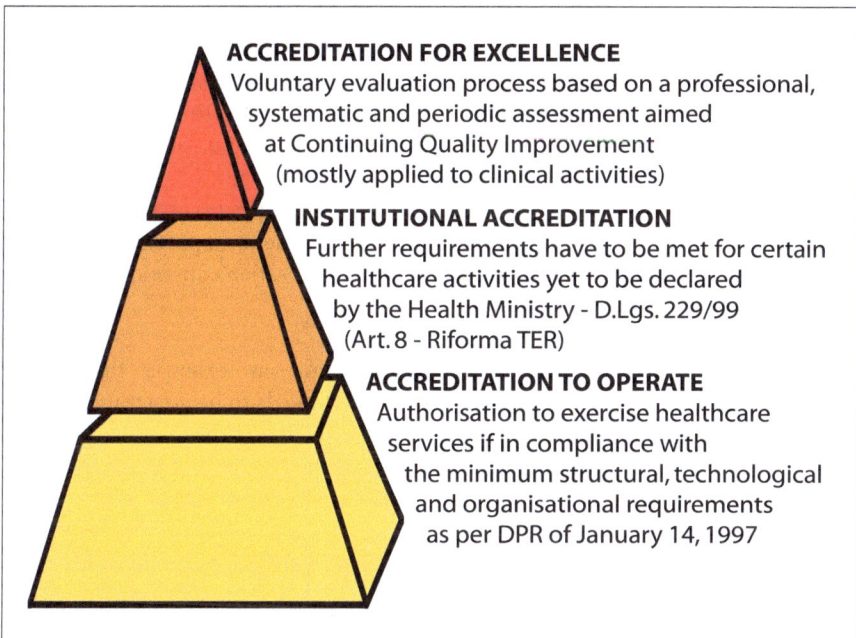

ACCREDITATION FOR EXCELLENCE
Voluntary evaluation process based on a professional,
systematic and periodic assessment aimed
at Continuing Quality Improvement
(mostly applied to clinical activities)

INSTITUTIONAL ACCREDITATION
Further requirements have to be met for certain
healthcare activities yet to be declared
by the Health Ministry - D.Lgs. 229/99
(Art. 8 - Riforma TER)

ACCREDITATION TO OPERATE
Authorisation to exercise healthcare
services if in compliance with
the minimum structural, technological
and organisational requirements
as per DPR of January 14, 1997

Fig. 1. Accreditation criteria

tries. The CEN (European Committee for Standardisation) reorganised them to apply to the European context, while the UNI (the Italian Agency for Standardisation) translated them and introduced them in Italy.

The ISO 9000 norms are subject to periodic revision. They were first published in 1987, revised in 1994 and again in 2000, resulting in the publication of UNI EN ISO 9001:2000, better known as "Vision 2000".

The ISO 9001:2000 model outlines what is required for the establishment of a Quality Management System, i.e. the complete and often complex organisation necessary for the management of a Quality-oriented company. This concept is of great interest to the healthcare world, since institutions such as the local healthcare units (ASL) and hospitals are taking on organisational structures and rules more and more similar to those of private companies.

The new norms, i.e. "Vision 2000", not only emphasise "Quality control and assurance", but also "planning and improvement". The new model aims to help organisations address fundamental needs, from the perspective of a "Quality Management System", focusing attention on the processes and how they are managed.

The norms of the new ISO 9000 series are:

- UNI EN ISO 9000:2000 "Quality Management System – Fundamentals and Terminology" UNI Milan 2000, which outlines the basic terminology regarding the concepts related to Quality, thus facilitating communication and understanding on an international level.
- UNI EN ISO 9001:2000 "Quality Management System – Requirements" UNI Milan 2000, which outlines the norms for certification, i.e. rules and models that equate to the minimum requirements for certification. Additionally, it out-

lines the management and resource base which has to be in place to efficiently establish and maintain the Quality Management System. The UNI EN ISO 9001:2000 focuses the organisation's attention on the system's efficacy. The model can thus be applied by the healthcare organisation that intends to show its customers-users its capability of guaranteeing a regular product and regularly monitored services, thus increasing satisfaction.

- UNI EN ISO 9004:2000 "Quality Management System – Guidelines for Performance Improvement" UNI Milan 2000. A guide to improving the Quality Management System, focusing the healthcare organisation's attention on the system's performance.

If a healthcare organisation, or a specific unit, for example the Unit of Pneumology, aims to obtain official recognition, it needs to be structured, organised and to operate in accordance with the specific norms of UNI EN ISO 9001:2000. This will underline its adherence to the norms (and obviously the law) and the related quality standards. This recognition is known in the international arena as "third-party certification".

The ISO 9000 norms, following the third-party certification methodology, go a step further from norms based on self-certification (first-party certification) and/or customer-user-based certification which is not always objective (second-party certification).

The third party, responsible for verifying the organisation's compliance to the Quality Management System and the ISO 9001:2000 requirements, is an independent party (such as CERTICHIM-CERTIQUALITY, IMQ-CSQ, TÜV, BSI, DNV), and more specifically in Italy it is an association or organisation working both at a national and international level and authorised by SINCERT (National System for the Accreditation of Certification Agencies).

The Quality Management System certification is obtained by demonstrating to the interested parties that the quality approach has been followed as regards management activities.

Thus, not only is there a well-described and documented management system, but, more importantly, processes and responsibilities have been outlined and defined within the organisation and the organisation pursues established and measurable objectives, aimed at the continuing improvement of products and services.

The ISO 9001:2000 Model and Its Relevance to Pneumology

The new model aims to help organisations answer the fundamental needs of a Quality Management System, focusing attention on the processes and their governance (Fig. 2).

The UNI EN ISO 9001:2000 describes the Quality Management System by representing it as a cycle aimed at "Continuing Quality Improvement" of services. The circular nature of the system is held together by four "macro processes":

- Responsibilities at the managerial level
- Resource management
- Processes occurring within the organisation, in this case the Unit of

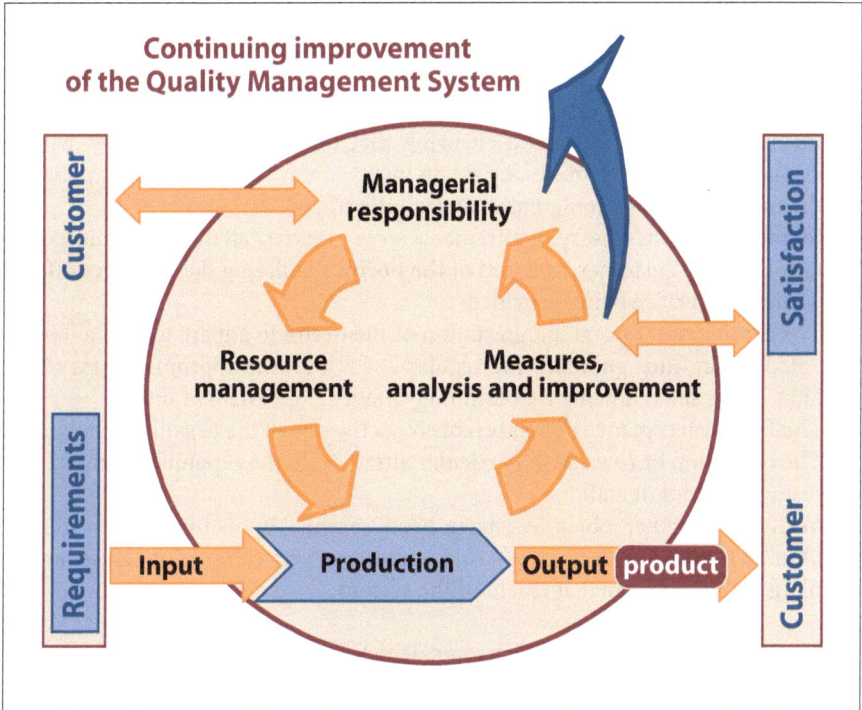

Fig. 2. The Quality Management System described by UNI EN ISO 9001:2000

Pneumology and more specifically home-based oxygen therapy
* Measures, analysis and improvement

Therefore, if the activity of each "operator" within the Unit, whether simple or complex, is focused on the consistent accomplishment of positive results as regards the deontological abidance of rules in the interest of patients' health, then the Quality Management System is nothing more than a good aid to the realisation of objectives.

The Quality Management System is not different to the usual operational system, but rather it is its representation and the model to be used for the management of both the operational and organisational activities, so as to guarantee that the services offered are in accordance with the needs of the client and the available resources.

This system is a useful aid in pinpointing the critical processes within a Pneumology Unit, allowing for purposeful and functional intervention in a specific phase of activities whether linked to one's own performance or the services being offered.

In our case it has given us the opportunity to consistently carry out home-based oxygen therapy within our area of competence in pneumology, in full accordance with the national and regional rules and following the standards laid out by the guidelines issued by scientific societies.

The ISO 9001:2000 organisational model, applied to pneumology, adheres to the four following chapters.

The *Responsibilities at a Managerial Level* chapter, which defines the objectives and how they can be reached:

- Participation at a managerial level, so as to explicitly guarantee managers' involvement in planning and ensuring that the necessary resources will be available to fulfil the aims being set. In our case this was specifically applied to the management of home-based oxygen therapy.
- Identifying the necessary requirements so as to satisfy all the needs and expectations of the customer-user and of the norms regulating the activities offered within the service being provided.
- The explicit and formal manifestation of the desire to adhere to a Quality-oriented policy, thus guaranteeing regular check-ups, the appropriateness of the aims being set, following a Continuing Quality Improvement line.
- The formal acceptance of measurable objectives at all the organisational levels.
- The definition of roles, with particular attention to the capabilities and related responsibilities of staff.
- Verifying whether objectives have been reached by examining the results obtained, and if necessary offering corrective, preventative or improvement plans to better the management of the system.

The *Resource Management* chapter, which requires identifying the means available and the necessary resources to obtain customer-user satisfaction by:

- The availability of adequate resources: company directives, development of new activities, new infrastructures, human resources (training, capabilities testing).

The *Product and/or Service Production* chapter, which relates to all the processes that are necessary to guarantee that the product or service reaches the customer-user, i.e. by:

- Planning the steps necessary to guarantee the services being offered (in our case the steps related to home-based oxygen therapy, where the primary service is the oxygen and the secondary services are all the activities needed to provide it).
- The processes related to the customer-user, i.e. identifying the customers' needs, analysing one's own operational capabilities aiming to satisfy their needs.
- Resource supply, etc.

The *Measures, Analysis and Improvement* chapter, to guarantee that the processes required for the product-service output are in line with the clients requests, by:

- Measuring and monitoring the services and final products being offered as well as customer satisfaction.
- Internal inspection (AUDIT).
- Management of the non-conformities in the service or product being offered (e.g. late presentation of the product, adverse events, insufficient supplies).
- Statistical data analysis to monitor the efficiency of the management system, using specific Quality indicators for each type of service offered, so as to plan preventative or corrective actions to ensure continuing improvement.

Process Approach and Management as a Basis for the Organisation of a Home-Based Oxygen Therapy Service

In the last few years a number of ISO 9001:2000 models have been used in the Italian healthcare system. Despite the fact that the application of these models was initially rare, today the possibility of its use not only in single operative units (as in our case with pneumology) but in the whole healthcare system is much stronger.

To facilitate the homogeneous connection between the pneumology unit and its related healthcare structure on a national level, the role of scientific societies is fundamental. So much so that the AIPO (Italian Association of Hospital Pneumologists) today has an ISO 9001:2000 certified Quality Management System, as regards the strategic processes that were outlined for 2004-2005.

For the single pneumology unit, independent of the accreditation models chosen by the related healthcare structure, there are a number of organisational principles which must be known and applied so as to obtain a home-based oxygen therapy capable of guaranteeing "assistance value" to the user and his/her family. These principles are:
- Process approach.
- Process management.

Attention to the client, leadership, staff involvement, process approach and management, decision-making based on facts, continuing improvement and mutually beneficial relationship with providers (source: ISO 9000:2000): These principles lead to a high performance and service based on Quality.

More specifically, the two principles most helpful in the management of home-based oxygen therapy are:

The *fourth principle*, "the process-based approach", which maintains that "a desired result is obtained more efficiently when the relative resources and activities are managed as a unit of related and interactive activities which transform the input elements into output elements".

The process is the sequence of related and interactive activities aimed at a specific final result, i.e. the output (Fig. 3). In this case, the process is oxygen therapy.

A first step is to describe the entire process from acceptance of the client's request

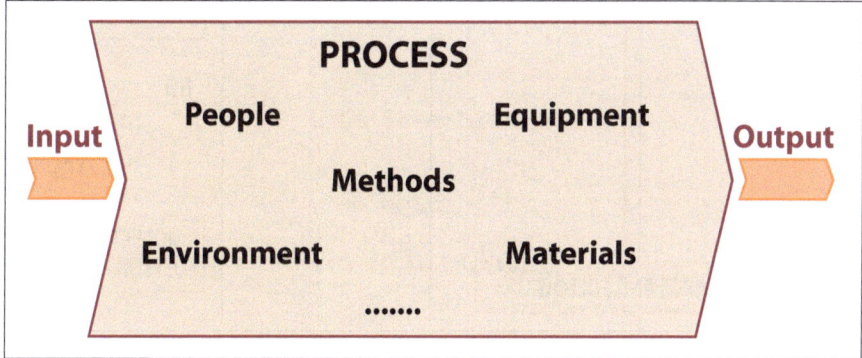

Fig. 3. A representation of "process"

(input) to the ultimate result (output), defining responsibilities, procedures, protocols etc. Figure 4 depicts a graphic representation of the oxygen therapy process.

The meaning of output is related to the added value generated by the process itself: the latter's value is higher when the quality and service capability (judged by the customer-user) is high and if it takes place with lower costs and in a shorter time span (judged by the organisation).

Furthermore, it is of fundamental importance to also manage all the related activities/responsibilities so as to enable a complete governance of the entire process. In the case of oxygen therapy, one must remember the "value chain", for example, the importance of a strong collaborative effort with the external oxygen provider as

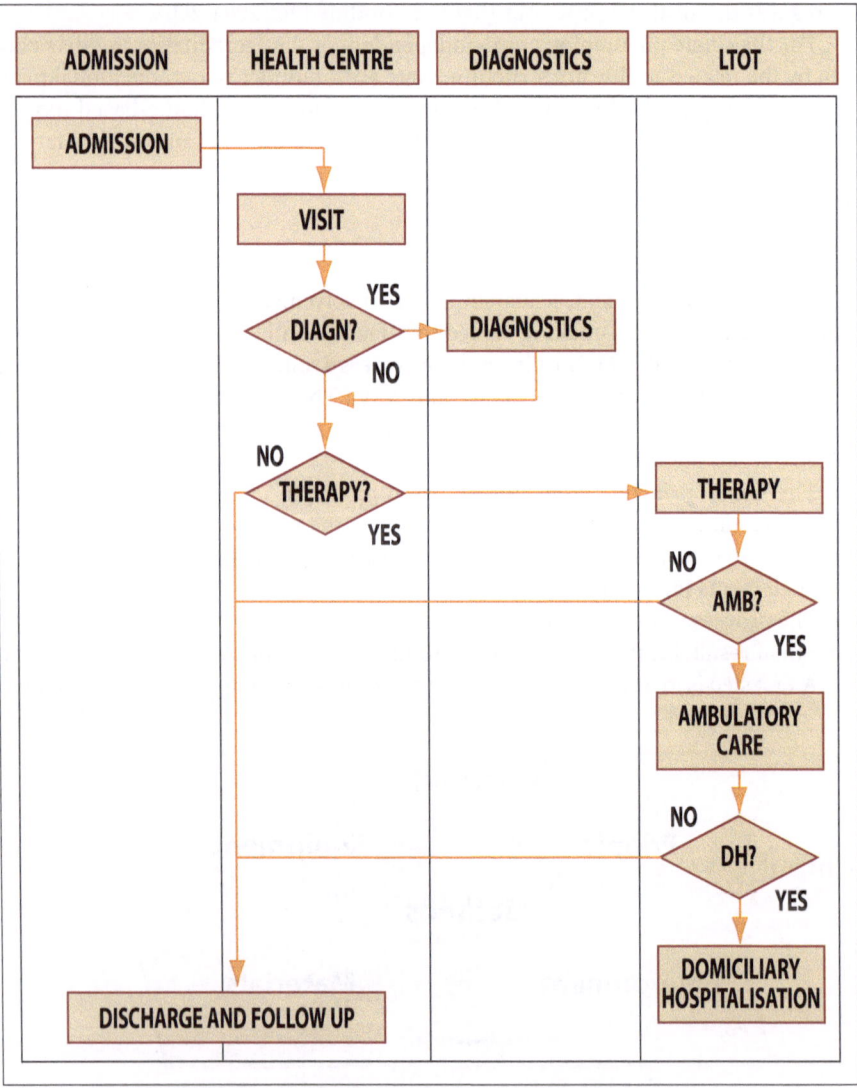

Fig. 4. A visual representation of the decision-making process for home-based oxygen therapy

regards the quality of the product and timing in changing the oxygen cylinders.

The other principle we need to emphasise is the *fifth one*, i.e. process management, which stresses that "identifying, understanding and managing a system of interconnected processes to obtain certain objectives contributes both to the efficiency and efficacy of the organisation".

Understanding the process clarifies the aims and objectives for all the operators involved, whereas the lack of clarity as regards the final aim of the process causes the staff to carry out their particular activity with different objectives. Process management results in a better understanding of the roles and responsibilities of the staff and thus allows the aims and objectives of the process and

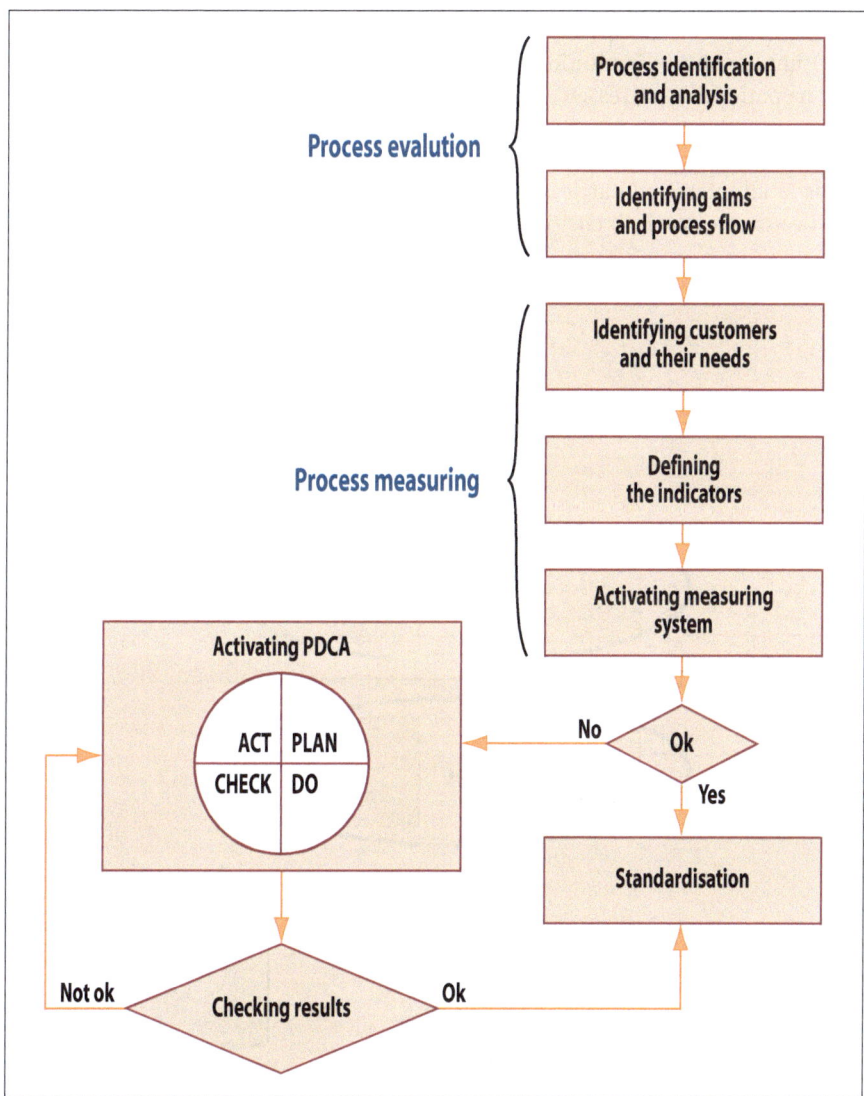

Fig. 5. Measuring processes as a first step to improvement

desired goals to be reached.

It is particularly important that the Pneumology Unit finds the instruments and methods to identify the performance and service indicators. The measuring phase follows the analysis of the process (Fig. 5) and requires that the Pneumology Unit is capable of monitoring the product/service characteristics, to verify whether they lie within the set standards. This activity has to be carried out when the production phase has been defined and used on a daily basis.

The process-measuring activities refer to the identification of the "clients" and their needs. In the case of oxygen therapy these are:
- The home-based patient
- The hospitalised patient
- The doctors of the operative units within the hospital
- Other healthcare institutions
- The patient's relatives, etc.

Providing a high-quality oxygen therapy service requires identification of the needs of all interested parties; this is the basis of the definition of an "indicator". The healthcare service's customer-users are the patients, and their perception of

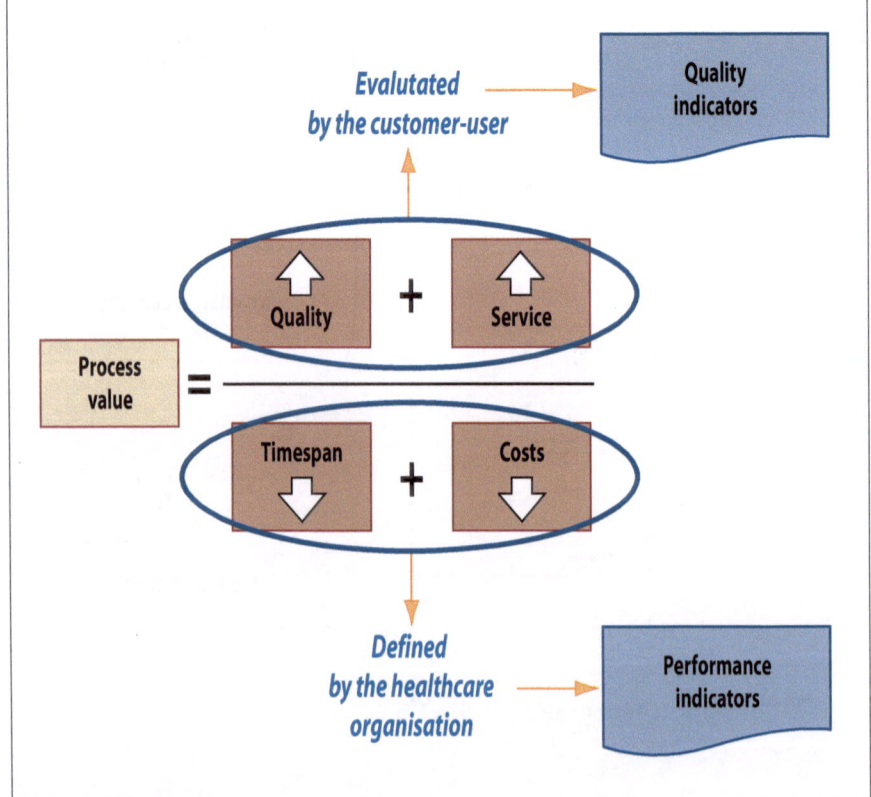

Fig. 6. Quality and performance indicators

Table 1. Two examples of indicators of telemetric LTOT performance monitored in severe (GOLD 3-4) COPD during a triennial LTOT programme: (A) the burden of *Pseudomonas aeruginosa* colonisation (*); (B) number of admissions/year due to pneumonia

	2001	2002	2003
A	31/141	29/151	27/133
	21.9%	19.2%	20.3%
(*) Chronic colonisation: *Pseudomonas aeruginosa* isolated from ≥80% of cultures for 3 years			
B	12/141	8/151	10/133
	8.5%	5.3%	7.5%

the service is one of the "Quality indicators". In this case, the performance evaluation tools consist of the match "Quality + service", and we can truly talk of performance indicators.

As mentioned above, there are other interested parties in the healthcare service, not only the customer-user. For example:

- The management level within the parent healthcare organisation
- The Pneumology Unit.

These types of customers, while respecting the expectations of the customer-user (i.e. the patient), are interested in evaluating the efficiency of the healthcare service provided. In this case, the efficiency indicators as well as the performance indicators are used. The value of the entire process is thus correlated with the performance and the quality indicators as represented in Fig. 6.

The indicators consist of the qualitative and quantitative information which is needed to evaluate the process over time and to verify that the objectives have been accomplished, thus allowing for an accurate decision-making process (Table 1).

As shown in Fig. 5, defining and collecting the indicators is the first step in the data analysis process, to guarantee the Quality monitoring of the service offered.

In conclusion, independent of the need of a structure to obtain the ISO 9001 certification, or whether it has to meet the regional, national or international accreditation standards, the application of basic principles such as the process approach and management in pneumology can guarantee the cultural growth of each operator and at the same time improve the healthcare system to safeguard positive results also in a risk management situation.

This is particularly true for home-based oxygen therapy, since the application of this system allows safeguarding of the customer-user and the relationship with relatives and viewing of these elements as the fundamental components to guarantee continuous assistance.

Suggested Reading

1. Barbarino FC (2002) Capire i processi. Come organizzarli, gestirli e migliorarli. UNI, Milan
2. Bizzarri G, Plebani M (2004) I processi del laboratorio clinico nell'ottica di sistema (ISO 9001:2000) dell'azienda sanitaria. Franco Angeli, Milan

3. Bosset LJ (1991) Quality function deployment. ASQC Quality Press, Milwaukee
4. Chakrapani C (1998) How to measure service quality & customer satisfaction. The informal field guide for tools and techniques. American Marketing Association, Chicago
5. Dal Negro R, Farina M (2005) (a cura di) L'approccio e la gestione per processi in pneumologia. Springer, Milan
6. Dal Negro R, Farina M (2003) L'applicazione pratica del modello ISO 9001:2000 in ambito pneumologico. Centro Scientifico Editore, Turin
7. Dal Negro R, Farina M (2002) Il modello ISO 9000 in pneumologia. Centro Scientifico Editore, Turin
8. Dal Negro R, Farina M (2001) La gestione per la qualità in Pneumologia. Aspetti applicativi secondo il modello ISO 9001:2000. Springer, Milan
9. Gramma A (1987) Gestire la qualità nei servizi. ISEDI, Turin
10. Leonardi E, (2000) Capire la qualità. Il Sole 24 Ore Libri, Milano
11. Leonardi E, Meacci S, Bergoglio R, Raiteri F, Bini S (2001) Conoscere le ISO 9000:2000. Cambiamento, cliente, processi e miglioramento continuo. UNI, Milan
12. Merli G, Biroli M (1996) Organizzazione e gestione per processi. ISEDI, Turin
13. Merli G (1999) I nuovi paradigmi del management. Il Sole 24 Ore, Milan
14. Oriani G (1995) Reengineering. Guerini e Associati, Milan
15. Pacchi C, Berti F, Di Stefano A, Natalucci G, Scarpetta M (2002) Qualità in organizzazioni sanitarie. FrancoAngeli, Milan
16. Tonchia S, Tramonatano A, Turchini S (2003) Gestione per processi e Knowledge management. Il Sole 24 Ore, Milan